Office Procedures for the Oral and Maxillofacial Surgeon

Editor

STUART E. LIEBLICH

ATLAS OF THE ORAL AND MAXILLOFACIAL SURGERY CLINICS OF NORTH AMERICA

www.oralmaxsurgeryatlas.theclinics.com

Consulting Editor
RICHARD H. HAUG

September 2013 • Volume 21 • Number 2

ELSEVIER

1600 John F. Kennedy Boulevard • Suite 1800 • Philadelphia, Pennsylvania, 19103-2899
http://www.oralmaxsurgeryatlas.theclinics.com

ATLAS OF THE ORAL AND MAXILLOFACIAL SURGERY CLINICS OF NORTH AMERICA Volume 21, Number 2
September 2013 ISSN 1061-3315 ISBN-13: 978-0-323-18844-9

Editor: John Vassallo; j.vassallo@elsevier.com
Development Editor: Susan Showalter

Reprints. For copies of 100 or more of articles in this publication, please contact the Commercial Reprints Department, Elsevier Inc., 360 Park Avenue South, New York, NY 10010-1710. Tel.: 212-633-3812; Fax: 212-462-1935; E-mail: reprints@elsevier.com.

Atlas of the Oral and Maxillofacial Surgery Clinics of North America (ISSN 1061-3315) is published biannually by Elsevier, 360 Park Avenue South, New York, NY 10010-1710. Months of issue are March and September. Periodicals postage paid at New York, NY and additional mailing offices. Subscription prices are $431.00 for international individual, $350.00 for US individual and Canadian individual; $210.00 for international student and Canadian student, $171.00 for US student; $434.00 for international institution and Canadian institution, $364.00 for US institution. Foreign air speed delivery is included in all *Clinics* subscription prices. All prices are subject to change without notice. POSTMASTER: Send address changes to *Atlas of the Oral and Maxillofacial Surgery Clinics of North America*, Health Sciences Division, Subscription Customer Service, 3251 Riverport Lane, Maryland Heights, MO 63043. Tel: 1-800-654-2452 (U.S. and Canada); 314-447-8871 (outside U.S. and Canada). Fax: 314-417-8029. E-mail: journalscustomerservice-usa@elsevier.com (for print support); journalsonline support-usa@elsevier.com (for online support).

Atlas of the Oral and Maxillofacial Surgery Clinics of North America is covered in *MEDLINE/PubMed (Index Medicus)*.

Printed and bound by CPI Group (UK) Ltd, Croydon, CR0 4YY

Transferred to digital print 2013

Contributors

CONSULTING EDITOR

RICHARD H. HAUG, DDS
Carolinas Center for Oral Health, Charlotte, North Carolina

EDITOR

STUART E. LIEBLICH, DMD
Private Practice, Avon Oral and Maxillofacial Surgery, Avon, Connecticut; Associate Clinical Professor, Department of Oral and Maxillofacial Surgery, University of Connecticut School of Dental Medicine, Farmington, Connecticut; Visiting Assistant Professor, Tufts University School of Dental Medicine, Boston, Massachusetts

AUTHORS

TYLER BOYNTON, DMD
Resident, Department of Oral and Maxillofacial Surgery, University of Connecticut School of Dental Medicine, Farmington, Connecticut

CHRISTOPHER CHOI, DDS, MD
Private Practice, Inland Empire Oral and Maxillofacial Surgeons, Rancho Cucamonga, California; Former Fellow, Carolinas Center for Oral and Facial Surgery, Charlotte, North Carolina

HARRY DYM, DDS
Chairman, Department of Dentistry and Oral and Maxillofacial Surgery, The Brooklyn Hospital Center, Brooklyn, New York

MARK C. FLETCHER, DMD, MD
Avon Oral and Maxillofacial Surgery, Avon, Connecticut

JACOB GADY, DMD, MD
Resident, Department of Craniofacial Sciences, Division of Oral and Maxillofacial Surgery, University of Connecticut School of Dental Medicine, Farmington, Connecticut

DANIEL GILL, DDS, MD
Chief Resident, Department of Oral and Maxillofacial Surgery, University of Connecticut School of Dental Medicine, Farmington, Connecticut

MARTIN L. GONZALEZ, MS
Senior Research Associate, American Association of Oral and Maxillofacial Surgeons, Rosemont, Illinois

REGINALD E. GOWANS, DDS
Assistant Professor, Charles R. Drew University, Los Angeles, California

RICHARD D. LEATHERS, DDS
Adjunct Assistant Professor, Division of Oral and Maxillofacial Surgery, UCLA School of Dentistry, Harbor UCLA Medical Center, Torrance, California

STUART E. LIEBLICH, DMD
Private Practice, Avon Oral and Maxillofacial Surgery, Avon, Connecticut; Associate Clinical Professor, Department of Oral and Maxillofacial Surgery, University of Connecticut School of Dental Medicine, Farmington, Connecticut; Visiting Assistant Professor, Tufts University School of Dental Medicine, Boston, Massachusetts

STANLEY LIU, DDS, MD
OMFS Resident, Department of Oral and Maxillofacial Surgery, University of California at San Francisco, San Francisco, California

CHIRAG PATEL, DMD, MD
OMFS Resident, Department of Oral and Maxillofacial Surgery, University of California at San Francisco, San Francisco, California

RICHARD C. ROBERT, DDS, MS
Clinical Professor, Department of Oral and Maxillofacial Surgery, University of California at San Francisco, San Francisco; Oral and Maxillofacial Surgery, San Francisco, California

SALVATORE L. RUGGIERO, DMD, MD, FACS
Clinical Professor, Division of Oral and Maxillofacial Surgery, Hofstra North Shore/LIJ School of Medicine, Hempstead, New York; Department of Oral and Maxillofacial Surgery, Stony Brook School of Dental Medicine, Stony Brook, New York

KEITH SHERWOOD, DDS
Associate Professor, Department of Orthodontics, Goldman School of Dental Medicine, Boston University, Boston, Massachusetts; Medical Staff and Chief, Department of Oral and Maxillofacial Surgery, Beverly Hospital, Beverly, Massachusetts

DANIEL SPAGNOLI, DDS, MS, PhD
Associate Professor and Chairman, Department of Oral and Maxillofacial Surgery, LSU HSC School of Dentistry, Louisiana State University, New Orleans, Louisiana

JOSHUA WOLF, DDS
Resident, Department of Oral and Maxillofacial Surgery, The Brooklyn Hospital Center, Brooklyn, New York

Contents

ATLAS OF THE ORAL AND MAXILLOFACIAL SURGERY CLINICS OF NORTH AMERICA

THE CLINICS ARE NOW AVAILABLE ONLINE!

Access your subscription at:
www.theclinics.com

Preface

Office Procedures for the Oral and Maxillofacial Surgeon

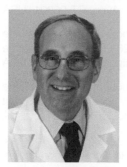

Stuart E. Lieblich, DMD
Editor

It gives me great pleasure to have the role as editor of this issue of the *Atlas of the Oral and Maxillofacial Surgery Clinics of North America*. Our profession has a rich depth and breadth of knowledge and surgical procedures that are utilized for the betterment of our patients. Although many complex procedures require management of cases in a hospital setting, most practitioners have a robust office practice. In that regard, this issue presents some valuable insights in the care of patients that present to our offices.

The office-based practice fulfills an important role in the health care system. However, there is a potential for the practitioner to abandon the hospital setting due to concerns with having to take trauma calls, the need to attend committee meetings, and the lower reimbursement of hospital cases. This was addressed in an editorial by Hupp in 2005.[1] I know I speak for all the authors of this issue that an active office-based practice does not prohibit one from maintaining an active hospital practice as well. Major surgical cases are an important component to our full scope of practice and I urge our colleagues to maintain hospital privileges. The American Board of Oral and Maxillofacial Surgery requires hospital privileges for the continuation of board certification (Certification Maintenance) as well, recognizing that our field is not a one-dimensional aspect.

I thank the authors of this issue for taking the time to share their expertise in the practice of oral and maxillofacial surgery. Their writing, as well as the extensive clinical pictures, depicts the concepts in an educational and interesting manner. It is a true commitment to our specialty that so many of the names you recognize are experts in our field, but just as exciting are the talents of their younger colleagues that collaborated with them on the articles. Our specialty is a vibrant one with a great continuity.

Certainly a vital aspect of the field of office-based procedures is the provision of outpatient anesthesia. Many patients are able to have care in the office setting that otherwise could not be completed. It therefore is fitting to have the opening article of this volume on that subject. I thank Dr Robert and his colleagues for the thorough review and highlighting of advancements in both anesthetic medications and also techniques for managing the airway.

Sharing his vast expertise on the diagnosis and management of osteonecrosis is Dr Ruggiero. This problem is one that has been recognized by the OMFS and brought to the attention of the medical community as a side effect from specific medications. We all face patients with this issue in our practices and they look to us for the management of this issue.

Then we get to the teeth. Drs Spagnoli and Choi provide a contemporary solution to the loss of important structural and esthetic aspects of the extraction socket with the use of rBMP. Drs Leathers and Gowans review the management of dentoalveolar trauma discussing the emergent care of this specific type of injury. We are fortunate to have the contribution of an orthodontist and OMFS, Dr Keith Sherwood, to provide an evidence-based approach to the orthodontic management

Atlas Oral Maxillofacial Surg Clin N Am 21 (2013) vii–viii
1061-3315/13/$ - see front matter © 2013 Elsevier Inc. All rights reserved.
http://dx.doi.org/10.1016/j.cxom.2013.06.002

of impacted teeth. Some impacted teeth present outside the "norm" of what we all see in our day-to-day practices. Drs Wolf and Dym review and illustrate these unusual impactions and offer salient suggestions for management.

Leaning heavily on local knowledge here in Connecticut, we have a section that describes and well documents the technique for coronectomy procedures by Drs Gady and Fletcher. I also had the privilege of working directly on two articles with our residents, Drs Gill and Boynton, who wrote on skeletal anchorage techniques and surgical uprighting of second molars. Again these are all procedures that we hope you can integrate into your practice with excellent results.

I want to take the privilege of dedicating this issue to my family: my parents, Severyn and Phyllis Lieblich, my mother-in-law, Edna Bente, and my late father-in-law Paul Bente Jr. As I write this on the day before Father's Day and on the "cusp" of my 30th wedding anniversary, I am so blessed to have two wonderful children, Brett and Margot, and to share this with my wife, colleague, companion, and soul mate, Janot Bente, DMD. I have so much to be thankful for that a brief line or two doesn't do justice. I have looked to all of you for your inspiration and guidance and you have always been there.

Stuart E. Lieblich, DMD
Avon Oral and Maxillofacial Surgery
34 Dale Road
Suite 105
Avon, CT 06001, USA

University of Connecticut School of Dental Medicine
263 Farmington Avenue
Farmington, CT 06030, USA

Tufts University School of Dental Medicine
One Kneeland Street
Boston, MA 02111, USA

E-mail address:
SLieblich@avonomfs.com

Reference

1. Hupp JR. Retreating to our cottages. Oral Surg Oral Med Oral Pathol Oral Radiol Endod 2005;99:391–3.

Advancements in Office-Based Anesthesia in Oral and Maxillofacial Surgery

Richard C. Robert, DDS, MS [a,b,]*, Stanley Liu, DDS, MD [a], Chirag Patel, DMD, MD [a], Martin L. Gonzalez, MS [c]

KEYWORDS

- Infusion • Pump • LMA • Laryngeal • Mask • Airway • Capnography

KEY POINTS

- An infusion pump enables delivery of a smooth anesthetic consisting of propofol or propofol combined with other rapid-onset/offset agents such as ketamine and remifentanil.
- Maintenance intravenous therapy during anesthesia for oral and maxillofacial surgery (OMS) should consist of an isotonic crystalloid solution such as normal saline or lactated Ringer 15 mL/Kg and intravenous access with an angiocatheter as opposed to a metal needle.
- For patients at risk for postoperative nausea and vomiting, a multimodal approach should be used with agents that are antagonists at $5-HT_3$, dopamine 2, and muscarinic receptors augmented by dexamethasone and propofol as an anesthetic.
- Obese patients with obstructive sleep apnea and gastroesophageal reflux disease represent an airway risk for which airway adjuncts such as a laryngeal mask airway, nasopharyngeal catheter, or tongue suture should be considered.
- Capnography and pretracheal auscultation with a Bluetooth pretracheal stethoscope provide essential monitoring of ventilation during office-based anesthesia.

Introduction

It is fitting that the first decade of a new millennium would witness significant advancements in office-based anesthesia in oral and maxillofacial surgery (OMS). These advancements are numerous and far reaching, and include the agents most commonly used and their method of delivery, as well as perioperative management and monitoring. In this article, some of the more significant of these advancements that have taken place during the last decade are explored. A useful tool in monitoring the changes has been the benchmark studies conducted by the American Association of Oral and Maxillofacial Surgeons (AAOMS). The first of these studies was fielded at the beginning of the last decade and the current one at the beginning of the second, in 2011 to 2012. The first study[1] relied on volunteers and took place over several years, with a cohort of nearly 25,000 patients. Participants in the second study were chosen by a random sampling. The preliminary data from this latter study are just becoming available and currently consist of a cohort of approximately 2600 patients. Because the data from the current registry are preliminary and there are

differences in study design, only general comparisons can be made to monitor trends (Table 1).

Comparison of the data from the 2 AAOMS studies (see Table 1) shows that third molar removal continues to be the most frequently performed procedure (approximately 70%). On the other hand, over the decade, other dentoalveolar procedures have decreased by more than 50% ($P<.001$), whereas implant procedures have increased 50% ($P<.001$). The operating surgeon continues to be the primary manager of anesthesia, and nearly 90% of the procedures performed are less than an hour in length. However, the 2011 to 2012 study suggests that there is an increase of more than 30% in procedures greater than 30 minutes in length ($P<.001$), which may in part be a reflection of the increase in implant procedures.

Agents

Primary Intravenous Anesthetic Agents

The modern era of office-based anesthesia in our specialty began in the 1950s, when Hubbell and Krogh popularized the use of intravenous (IV) Pentothal (thiopental) anesthesia. Pentothal was replaced by the shorter-acting barbiturate methohexital, which continued to be the primary agent used for office-based anesthesia until the end of the century. However, when problems developed at the production facility for methohexital in the early years of the twenty-first century, many surgeons were forced to turn to propofol, which had largely replaced the barbiturates in medical anesthesia during the previous decade. Although methohexital returned to the marketplace, many of those oral and maxillofacial surgeons

Disclosures: The authors have nothing to disclose.

[a] Department of Oral and Maxillofacial Surgery, University of California at San Francisco, San Francisco, CA, USA
[b] Oral and Maxillofacial Surgery, 2400 Westborough Boulevard, Suite 211, San Francisco, CA 94080, USA
[c] American Association of Oral and Maxillofacial Surgeons, Rosemont, IL, USA
* Corresponding author. Department of Oral and Maxillofacial Surgery, University of California at San Francisco, San Francisco, CA.
E-mail address: RCR2400@aol.com

Atlas Oral Maxillofacial Surg Clin N Am 21 (2013) 139–165
1061-3315/13/$ - see front matter © 2013 Elsevier Inc. All rights reserved.
http://dx.doi.org/10.1016/j.cxom.2013.05.007

Table 1 The patients, providers, and perioperative management of the AAOMS benchmark studies

	Data from 2000[a]	Data from 2011–2012[b]	% Change	P Value
Number of Patients	24,737	2577		
Procedure Performed				
Third molar	16,892 (68.3%)	1834 (71.2%)	↑ 4.2%	<.003
Other dentoalveolar	17,652 (30.9%)	566 (22.0%)	↓ 53.1%	<.0001
Implant	650 (2.6%)	101 (3.9%)	↑ 50.0%	<.0001
Primary Manager of Anesthesia				
Operating surgeon	23,576 (95.5%)	2410 (93.5%)	↓ 2.1%	<.0001
Certified registered nurse anesthetist	654 (2.6%)	88 (3.4%)	↑ 30.8%	<.03
Anesthesia Time (min)				
10–30	14,622 (59.1%)	1216 (47.2%)	↓ 20.1%	<.0001
31–60	7588 (30.7%)	1042 (40.4%)	↑ 31.6%	<.0001
IV Access Device				
Straight needle or butterfly	12,218 (49.4%)	430 (16.6%)	↓ 66.4%	<.0001
Angiocatheter	12,313 (49.8%)	2124 (82.4%)	↑ 65.5%	<.0001
IV Fluids				
None used	9208 (37.2)	0	↓ 100%	<.0001
IV fluids used	15,529 (62.8)	2555 (99.2)	↑ 50.0%	<.000

[a] Published in *J Oral Maxillofac Surg* 2003;61(9):988.
[b] Unpublished preliminary data.
Courtesy of Martin L. Gonzalez, MS, Senior Research Associate, American Association of Oral and Maxillofacial Surgeons, Rosemont, IL.

who had begun using propofol no longer wished to return to methohexital. Data from the AAOMS benchmarking studies (Table 2) indicate that most (approximately 70%; $P<.002$) patients receive propofol as their primary anesthetic agent. However, at the time of the first study a decade ago, a virtually identical large majority (approximately 70%; $P<.001$) were receiving methohexital and only approximately 20% were receiving propofol.

Two of the primary characteristics that have made propofol so popular with anesthesiologists and oral and maxillofacial surgeons are its rapid onset and offset.[2] The rapid onset is largely caused by its chemical structure (Fig. 1). First, the molecule is small, which allows easy passage through the blood-brain barrier (Fig. 2). The second characteristic is its high lipoid solubility and its resistance to its ionization. As a so-

called hindered phenol, the hydroxyl radical of propofol at carbon 1 is protected from ionization by the bulky isopropyl groups at carbons 2 and 6 (see Fig. 1). The offset of propofol is caused by both rapid redistribution and rapid metabolism. Historically, the parameter of elimination half-life ($T_{\frac{1}{2}\beta}$) has not adequately accounted for both the rapid redistribution and biotransformation, which are in turn responsible for the rapid dissipation of the effects of such drugs as propofol. Consequently, a new parameter, the context-sensitive half-time, was developed and is described later.

Because its chemical structure provides propofol with rapid access to its receptor sites in the central nervous system (CNS), it can quickly bind to them and have a commensurate rapid onset. However, the bond is short-lived, and soon the propofol molecules return to the central circulation and pass to other

Table 2 The anesthetic agents and ancillary drugs received by patients in the AAOMS benchmark studies

	Data from 2000[a]	Data from 2011–2012[b]	% Change	P Value
Primary Parental Drug Used				
Ketamine HCl	5284 (21.4%)	1187 (46.1%)	↑ 115.4%	<.0001
Methohexital	17,086 (69.1%)	285 (11.1%)	↓ 83.9%	<.0001
Propofol	4768 (19.3%)	1774 (68.8%)	↑ 256.5%	<.0001
Opioids Used				
Fentanyl	16,142 (65.3%)	1884 (73.1%)	↑ 11.9%	<.0001
Meperidine	3745 (15.1%)	77 (3.0%)	↓ 80.1%	<.0001
Remifentanil	0	156 (6.1%)		<.0001
Benzodiazepines Used				
Diazepam	5288 (21.4%)	62 (2.4%)	↓ 88.8%	<.0001
Midazolam	16,456 (66.5%)	2446 (94.9%)	↑ 42.7%	<.0001
Other Medications Used				
Dexamethasone	14,002 (56.6%)	1679 (65.2%)	↑ 15.2%	<.0001
Glycopyrrolate	5829 (23.6%)	720 (27.9%)	↑ 18.2%	<.0001

[a] Published in *J Oral Maxillofac Surg* 2003;61(9):987.
[b] Unpublished preliminary data.
Courtesy of Martin L. Gonzalez, MS, Senior Research Associate, American Association of Oral and Maxillofacial Surgeons, Rosemont, IL.

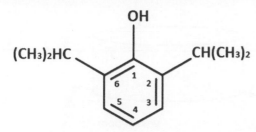

Fig. 1 The propofol formula. The molecule is a small one that rapidly passes through the blood-brain barrier. It is highly non-polarized because of isopropyl groups at carbons 2 and 6, which help prevent ionization of the hydroxyl group at carbon 1. (*Adapted from* Morgan GE, Mikhail MS, Murray MJ. Clinical anesthesiology. 4th edition. New York: Lange Medical Books/McGraw-Hill, Medical Pub. Division; 2006. p. 198, 1105; with permission.)

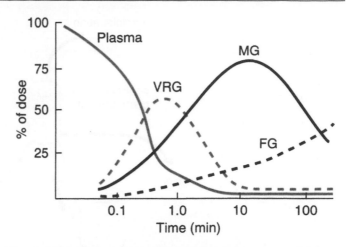

Fig. 3 Distribution of thiopental into the tissues of the body, including the vessel-rich group (VRG), the muscle group (MG), and the fat group (FG). (*From* Morgan GE, Mikhail MS, Murray MJ. Clinical anesthesiology. 4th edition. New York: Lange Medical Books/McGraw-Hill, Medical Pub. Division; 2006. p. 186, 1105; with permission.)

parts of the body in a manner similar to that of barbiturates (Fig. 3). However, not all of the body tissues have the same level of vascularity. Consequently, the tissues have been artificially divided into compartments based on their extent of vascularization. These compartments are shown in the model in Fig. 4 and include a central compartment, a vessel-rich compartment, a vessel-poor compartment, and an intermediate compartment. Once the propofol molecules have passed into the various compartments, they return to the central circulation and pass through the liver, where much of the biotransformation of the drug takes place. The biotransformed drug is eliminated through the urine. In addition, propofol has been shown to have extrahepatic metabolism, and elimination is in part through the lungs.

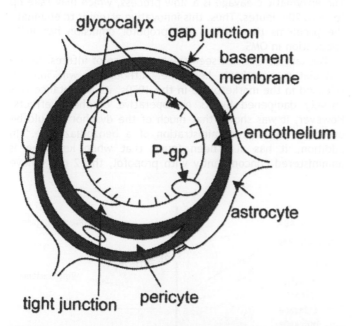

Fig. 2 Schema of the blood-brain barrier, which consists of polarized endothelial cells interconnected by complex tight junctions that limit paracellular permeability. In addition, the perivascular astrocyte end-feet almost totally cover the abluminal surface of the basement membrane. These characteristics allow the passage of only small molecules such as those of propofol. (*From* Ueno M. Mechanisms of the penetration of blood-borne substances into the brain. Curr Neuropharmacol 2009;7(2):143; with permission.)

The context-sensitive half-time was developed to take into account the complex fate of drugs such as propofol described earlier. It is based on calculations derived from the volumes of distribution of these drugs. These volumes represent the theoretical volume into which the drug is distributed, which in turn is based on the rapidity of that redistribution. The context-sensitive half-time is a computer-generated value that represents the time required for the concentration of the drug in the plasma to decrease to a level of 50% once an infusion of the drug has been discontinued. It is then a reflection of the pattern of the dissipation of drug affect. The context-sensitive half-time plot for several IV anesthetic agents is shown in Fig. 5. In general, those drugs that have a low, relatively flat plot are those that are associated with rapid dissipation of drug effect and the likelihood of early discharge for the patient. Thus, the more desirable plot of propofol can be appreciated when it is compared with the ultra—short-acting barbiturate agents thiopental and methohexital.

Another intriguing property of propofol is the manner in which it interacts with the γ-aminobutyric acid A (GABA$_A$) receptor. The GABA$_A$ receptor initially described for the benzodiazepines has proved to be the receptor for several anesthetic agents, including the barbiturates, propofol, etomidate, and inhalation agents (Fig. 6). The receptor is one of the most extensively studied and , has a familiar configuration, consisting of 2 α subunits, 2 β subunits, and a γ subunit. However, there are at least 3 subtypes of the β subunit, which have been designated β_1, β_2, and β_3 (Fig. 7). Those GABA$_A$ receptors that contain the β_3 subtype are those that are the target for high doses of propofol, which induce immobilization and general anesthesia. However, when propofol interacts with GABA$_A$ receptors that contain only β_1 and β_2 subtypes, it facilitates GABA in opening of the chloride channel in a manner similar to that which has long been associated with benzodiazepine action. This dual action of propofol is important from a clinical standpoint. Because of this characteristic, propofol can be used for deep sedation and general anesthesia at high doses and yet function as a sedative agent facilitating the action of GABA at lower doses. Thus, the agent has found a place in the sedation of older or medically compromised patients as well as those patients who are undergoing lengthy procedures such as implant or bone graft surgery.

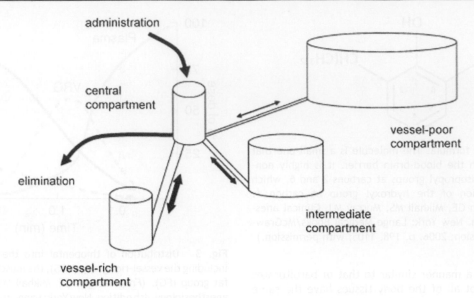

Fig. 4 A multicompartment model showing the dynamic passage of rapidly redistributing drugs among the various compartments and central circulation. (*From* Roberts F, Freshwater-Turner D. Pharmacokinetics and anesthesia. Cont Educ Anaesth Crit Care Pain 2007;7(1):26; with permission.)

Propofol also differs from the barbiturates in several other ways. In particular, it has antiemetic properties and provides an element of postoperative euphoria. It seems that the antiemetic effects are related to 5-HT$_3$ antagonism in the area postrema, the location of the chemoreceptor trigger zone. Although the mechanism for postoperative euphoria of propofol has not been clearly elucidated, initial studies suggest that it may be related to increased dopamine concentrations in the nucleus accumbens, the same locus for the generation of the pleasurable effects of recreational drugs.

Propofol is an exceptional drug that has virtually revolutionized outpatient anesthesia in medicine as well as OMS. However, like all drugs, it has its shortcomings, a principal one

being its insolubility in blood. In an attempt to overcome this shortcoming, medicinal chemists have developed a prodrug of propofol, which has been termed fospropofol. A phosphate monoester was added to the propofol molecule, which renders the compound water soluble. After injection of the fospropofol into the bloodstream, there is in vivo cleavage of the phosphate ester by alkaline phosphatases, resulting in the liberation of the propofol for expression of its anesthetic effects. The enzymatic cleavage is a slow process, which may take up to 15 to 20 minutes. Thus, this innovative attempt to eliminate the problems that attend the propofol emulsion has little application in OMS.

The last decade has seen the resurgence of interest in the dissociative anesthetic ketamine. Although it was initially released in the marketplace in the 1970s, its acceptance was initially dampened by its postoperative dysphoric effects. However, it was shown that much of the dysphoria could be overcome by prior administration of a benzodiazepine.[3] In addition, it has also been found that when ketamine is administered concomitantly with propofol, the 2 drugs have

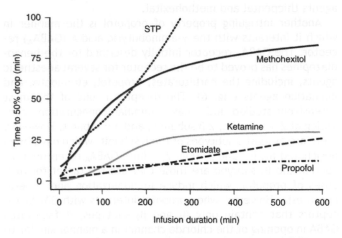

Fig. 5 The context-sensitive half-time plot of several IV anesthetic agents. Note the low, flat plot for propofol, which correlates closely with rapid recovery and readiness for discharge. (*Adapted from* Springman S. Ambulatory anesthesia: the requisites in anesthesiology. 1st edition. Philadelphia: Mosby; 2006, with permission; and Egan TD. Pharmacokinetics and rational intravenous drug selection and administration in anesthesia. In: Lake CI, Rice I, Sperry RJ, editors. Advances in anesthesia. vol. 12. St Louis (MO): Mosby; 1995. p. 38; with permission.)

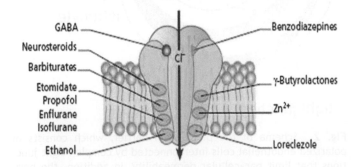

Fig. 6 There are several receptor sites for various anesthetic agents on the GABA$_A$ receptor. These sites include benzodiazepines, barbiturates, propofol, and inhalation agents. (*From* Evers SA, Maze M. Anesthetic pharmacology: physiologic principles and clinical practice. Philadelphia: Churchill Livingstone; 2004. p. 418; with permission.)

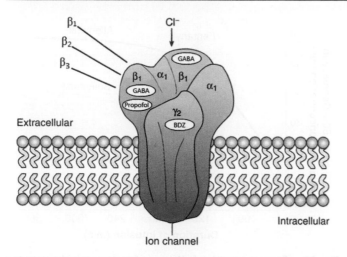

Fig. 7 The GABA_A receptor with its 2 α subunits, 2 β subunits, and 1 γ subunit. Note the 3 β subtypes β_1, β_2, and β_3, as described in the text. (*From* Miller RD. Miller's anesthesia. 7th edition. Philadelphia: Churchill Livingstone/Elsevier; 2010. p. 337; with permission.)

many desirable complementary effects. For instance, the tendency of ketamine to increase blood pressure counteracts the hypotensive effects of propofol. Although propofol causes respiratory depression and ketamine anesthesia is associated with minimal response to hypercapnia and provides significant bronchodilation, the postoperative euphoria provided by propofol augments the effects of the benzodiazepines in overcoming the dysphoric effects of ketamine. In addition, its context-sensitive half-time plot is similar to that of propofol (Fig. 8), which correlates closely with rapid recovery and readiness for discharge. Data from the AAOMS benchmark studies suggest that these desirable attributes of ketamine have led to inclusion of the drug in the approach of many surgeons to their office-based anesthetic. The current study indicates that approximately 46% of patients receive ketamine compared with only 21% in 2000 (see Table 2), an increase of approximately 115% (P<.001).

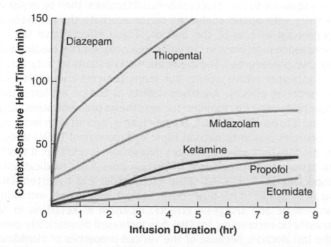

Fig. 8 Context-sensitive plot for several IV anesthetic agents showing the similar configuration of the propofol and ketamine plots. (*From* Hughes MA, Glass PS, Jacobs JR. Context-sensitive half-time in multicompartment pharmacokinetic models for IV anesthesia. Anesthesiology 1992;76:334–41; with permission.)

Preinduction Agents

Soon after the emergence of methohexital as a primary agent for office-based anesthesia in OMS, the first IV benzodiazepine diazepam was introduced by Leo Sternbach of Roche Laboratories. It became apparent that the inclusion of a benzodiazepine as a preinduction agent for methohexital anesthesia tended to smooth the course of the anesthetic. The phenylpiperidine synthetic opioid meperidine was added to provide the synergistic effects of a benzodiazepine/opioid combination. Over the next 2 to 3 decades, the combination of methohexital, diazepam, and meperidine gained wide acceptance. However, in the closing decades of the century, both a shorter-acting benzodiazepine and a new short-acting synthetic opioid became available. The shorter-acting benzodiazepine, midazolam, also had the desirable property of being water soluble, which significantly reduced the incidence of phlebitic complications associated with diazepam.[4] The shorter-acting synthetic opioid fentanyl, an anilidopiperidine, soon made inroads into many offices as well.

A comparison of the AAOMS studies (see Table 2) indicates that there has been a nearly 90% decrease (P<.001) in the number of patients receiving diazepam over the last decade. During the same decade, the percentage of patients receiving midazolam increased from approximately 66% to 95%, an increase of more than 40% (P<.001). That same decade has seen a decrease of approximately 80% (P<.001) in the number of patients receiving meperidine and an increase in the patients receiving fentanyl (see Table 2) from approximately 65% to 73%, an increase of approximately 12% (P<.001).

These trends suggest that meperidine is on its way out as a component of IV anesthesia in OMS. This trend in OMS reflects the attitude of the anesthetic community worldwide. The marked decline in the popularity of meperidine is based on several undesirable side effects. One of its primary metabolites, normeperidine, is only half as potent as meperidine as an analgesic but has two-thirds of its potency as a CNS excitatory agent. Furthermore, normeperidine has a long elimination half-life, which becomes particularly problematic in patients with renal disease. Its anticholinergic effects have been shown to lead to confusion as well as delirium and memory deficits, especially in the elderly. Because of these significant shortcomings, it is likely that the use of meperidine will continue to decrease.

The inclusion of benzodiazepines in a balanced IV anesthetic has had several desirable consequences. The benzodiazepines provide anxiolysis, sedation, and amnesia, which tend to make the IV anesthetic experience more comfortable for both the patient and the operator. There seem to be few downsides to their use, because they also cause little cardiorespiratory depression. However, there is growing concern that anesthesia in older patients may sometimes lead to delirium and cognitive dysfunction. Studies suggest that even short ambulatory procedures such as those that are common in OMS may be as likely a setting for these complications as general anesthesia. Benzodiazepines are viewed as a primary culprit. Because of these concerns, several prominent authorities in the field suggest that dosages of benzodiazepines should be markedly decreased or that benzodiazepines should be withheld altogether in the elderly. In the past, because of their presumed safety profile, benzodiazepines have played a prominent role in sedation for the elderly. It seems that a more reasonable alternative may be propofol in low, sedative doses.

Another concern in the use of preinduction and ancillary agents has been the respiratory depression that accompanies all opioid agents. This depression is of special concern in the sedation of both the elderly and of patients with morbid obesity and obstructive sleep apnea (OSA). Opioid-induced respiratory depression has been implicated in several fatalities. In these patient populations, markedly reduced dosages must be used and the use of nonopioid analgesics considered. An exciting innovation has been the introduction of the esterase-metabolized anilidopiperidine remifentanil (Fig. 9). Because esterases are found throughout all of the tissues of the body, enzymatic transformation of remifentanil is rapid and there is no wait for prolonged biotransformation in the liver.[5] This finding is mirrored in its low, flat plot of context-sensitive half-time (Fig. 10). However, the rapid offset of remifentanil introduces consideration of the use of an infusion pump for its administration, which is discussed later.

Anesthetic Premedications

During the last decades of the last century, oral anesthetic premedications for anxious patients usually consisted of relatively long-acting benzodiazepines such as diazepam. During the

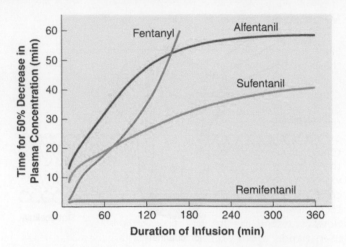

Fig. 10 Context-sensitive halftimes of various opioids. Note the low, flat plot for remifentanil, compared with the other opioids. (*From* Egan TD, Lemmens HJ, Fiset P, et al. The pharmacokinetics of the new short-acting opioid remifentanil (GI87084B) in healthy adult male volunteers. Anesthesiology 1993;79(5):881–92; with permission.)

first decade of the current century, diazepam was replaced in many practices by the shorter-acting benzodiazepine triazolam. After the initial release of the drug, isolated poorly substantiated reports of alleged tendency of triazolam to exacerbate suicidal tendencies caused much furor. It was shown that triazolam had the same safe track record as the other benzodiazepines. Consequently, the drug has become the favored drug for premedication in dentistry, including oral sedation for patients undergoing nonsurgical procedures by general dentists, periodontists, endodontists, and other practitioners who do not have training in general anesthesia. The medication has been used effectively as oral premedication in OMS. It comes in several strengths, including 0.125 mg, 0.25 mg, and 0.5 mg. Often, the 0.125-mg dose intended for geriatric patients is sufficient for premedications of younger patients as well.

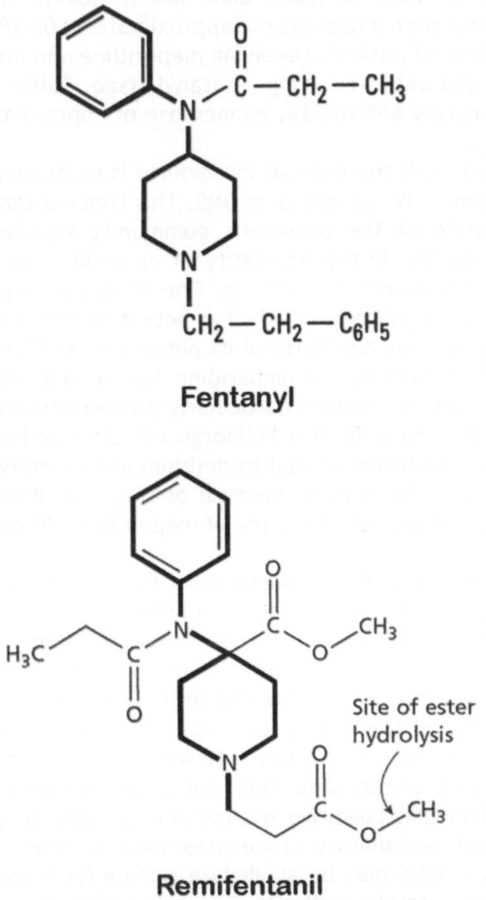

Although benzodiazepine premedication provides sedation and anxiolysis, even triazolam with its short duration of action can prolong recovery. In addition, in patients who are particularly sensitive to the effects of benzodiazepines, their synergistic activity with opioid analgesics can exacerbate the respiratory depressant effects of the opioids. These effects have led to resurgence in interest in clonidine as a preoperative medication for OMS procedures.[6] The medication was initially introduced as an antihypertensive agent, but many patients complained of its sedating effects. Anesthesiologists in Europe explored the possibility of using clonidine for anesthesia premedication, and found it to be efficacious. Clonidine is an α_2 agonist with sedative properties similar to natural rapid eye movement (REM) sleep, and it does not cause respiratory depression. In addition, it tends to attenuate the tendency of certain anesthetic medications, especially ketamine, to cause tachycardia and hypertension. As an α_2 agonist, it has other desirable qualities as well, including antiemetic and analgesic effects. Inclusion of ketamine in IV anesthetic techniques for OMS has increased dramatically over the last decade. Because of the various properties of clonidine discussed earlier, many surgeons have found that it provides an excellent premedication for patients who receive ketamine. In addition to providing sedation and counteracting the hypertensive and tachycardic effects of ketamine, it provides protection against the emetic effects of ketamine as well.

Fentanyl

Remifentanil

Fig. 9 Chemical formulas for fentanyl and remifentanil. Note the site of esterase hydrolysis of the ester moiety of remifentanil, which leads to its exceedingly rapid biotransformation by esterases throughout the body. (*From* Morgan GE, Mikhail MS, Murray MJ. Clinical anesthesiology. 4th edition. New York: Lange Medical Books/McGraw-Hill, Medical Pub. Division; 2006. p. 193, 1105; with permission.)

Medication delivery

Since its inception in the middle of the last century, IV anesthesia in OMS has been largely delivered by the so-called incremental bolus technique. Small increments of the various IV drugs are administered manually with syringes periodically during the procedure. Because of the more rapid dissipation of the effects of propofol compared with methohexital, the increments are usually smaller and more frequently administered. However, no incremental bolus technique can provide the same constant level of plasma concentration as that provided by an infusion pump. Initially, infusion pumps were cumbersome and complex, and it took several decades of technological advancements to overcome these shortcomings. However, within the last 2 decades less cumbersome and more user-friendly syringe-based infusion pumps have been developed. The most popular of these has been the Baxter Infuse O.R. syringe pump (Baxter Healthcare Corporation, Deerfield, IL, USA) (Fig. 11), which has found a home in outpatient surgery centers and hospitals throughout the country. It is a hybrid digital-analog device, which delivers a constant infusion through a syringe driven by an electronically controlled advancement screw. The device proved to be simple to program and provided reliable, constant drug delivery. However, 2 shortcomings of this type of infusion system have prompted Baxter to discontinue its production of the unit. In the modern era, new demands have been placed on infusion pumps. First,

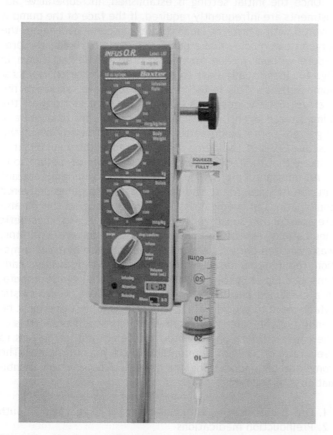

Fig. 11 The Baxter Infuse O.R. infusion pump, a hybrid analog-digital device. Although popular for many years amongst anesthetists and anesthesiologists, the device has no computer interface for the electronic medical record and no confirmation mode. It continues to be widely used in outpatient surgery centers and office-based anesthesia, but is no longer in production. (*Courtesy of* Richard C. Robert, DDS, MS, South San Francisco, CA.)

it must be possible for them to interface with a computer so that information from the pump can be incorporated into the electronic medical record. Second, pump-related complications have led to recommendations that pumps have a confirmation mode. This recommendation means that once a parameter for drug delivery (eg, rate of administration) has been entered into the pump, it must be confirmed by the anesthetist. The new pumps that have entered the market place are totally digital ones, which can interface with the electronic medical record and have a confirmation code.

Regardless of whether the operator delivers their IV anesthetic by an incremental bolus technique or with a pump, the object is to provide a constant blood level of the anesthetic agent. Over the last couple of decades, technologic improvements have made it possible for this goal to be accomplished with simple, easy-to-use infusion pumps, which have become almost universally accepted in hospitals and outpatient surgery centers. However, the long, ostensibly successful, track record of the incremental bolus technique in OMS has made most oral and maxillofacial surgeons reluctant to adopt the new technology. The number of oral and maxillofacial surgeons using infusion pumps is sufficiently low that use of a pump was not included in either of the AAOMS benchmark studies. However, unofficial polls conducted at anesthesia meetings suggest that an increasing number of oral and maxillofacial surgeons are beginning to use infusion pumps. With ever-increasing interest in rapid street readiness after office-based anesthesia with such drugs as propofol and remifentanil, infusion pumps are a logical choice. Medications such as propofol and remifentanil perform best when the receptors for these drugs are constantly bathed by the circulation of the agents in the bloodstream. Lapses in the plasma concentration lead to both patient movement and patient awareness, both of which are best minimized with an infusion pump.

Although infusion pumps for total IV anesthesia have been widely embraced by anesthesiologists, the few studies reporting on their use in the OMS literature have not shown an overwhelming difference in patient response to anesthetics delivered by an incremental bolus versus an infusion pump.[7] For an anesthetic model based on the delivery of anesthesia by the operating surgeon, a true double-blind study is virtually impossible to design. In those studies that have been performed, the difference between the 2 delivery techniques has been masked to some extent by the sedation and amnesia provided by preinduction administration of benzodiazepines and opioids. Furthermore, no studies have included balanced anesthetic techniques, in which propofol is combined with ketamine or remifentanil. Thus, further study in the application of infusion pumps for IV anesthesia in the OMS is warranted.

Modern infusion pumps incorporate considerable smart technology, which simplifies delivery of anesthetic agents. There are 2 syringe pumps that are most commonly purchased by oral and maxillofacial surgeons through equipment supply houses: the Medfusion 3500 (Smiths Medical, Dublin, OH, USA) (Fig. 12) and Aitecs 12S Pro (Aitechs-USA, Kernersville, NC, USA) (Fig. 13). Of the 2, the Medfusion pump has a more comprehensive drug library, and it has found a home in many hospitals and outpatient surgery centers. The Aitecs pump has a smaller drug library and fewer delivery options, but those available are more than adequate for the average OMS office. Consequently, our comments are addressed to the latter pump.

Before using an infusion pump, it is necessary for the operator to perform some simple steps, as shown in Figs. 13 and 14. In Fig. 1, loading of the syringe on the pump is shown.

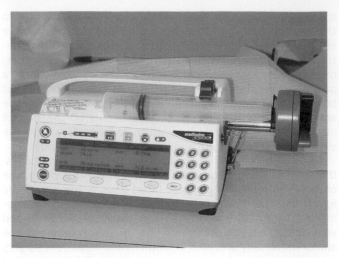

Fig. 12 The Medfusion 3500 infusion pump. The device has an extensive drug library and a wide variety of settings for drug delivery. (*Courtesy of* Richard C. Robert, DDS, MS, South San Francisco, CA.)

The pump is smart designed to sense the brand and size of the syringe (see Fig. 14). Plunger advancement is via a screw drive that is controlled by a digitally activated motor. There is a light-emitting diode (LED) window in the upper left-hand corner of the face of the pump, in which parameters are shown during the programming and operation of the pump. Nine parameters can be programmed, including the size of the syringe, the drug name (see Fig. 14), dosing mode, drug concentration, patient weight, infusion rate, bolus rate, bolus dose, and the occlusion level. Occlusion level represents the pressure that must build up in the line when it becomes occluded before the alarm sounds.

Several of the operating parameters can be set and left unchanged during pump operations. These parameters include the name of the drug, the dosing mode, concentration, and occlusion level. Parameters that must be set before pump operation for an individual patient include the patient's weight (see Fig. 14), infusion rate, bolus rate, and bolus dose. The latter 3 of these are determined by the gender, age, body

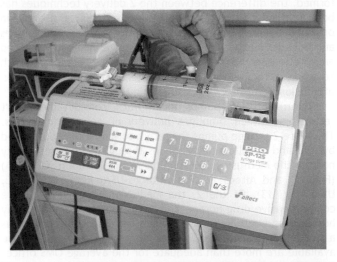

Fig. 13 The Aitecs Pro SP-12S infusion pump. Delivery of a constant infusion is via a syringe driven by an electronically controlled advancement screw. (*Courtesy of* Richard C. Robert, DDS, MS, South San Francisco, CA.)

habitus, and state of medical compromise of the patient. For instance, children require a higher infusion rate, bolus rate, and bolus dose than do teenagers and young adults. Conversely, lower settings should be established for geriatric patients and those who are medically compromised. It is also often helpful to program the pump such that the initial bolus (see Fig. 14) can be given in increments (usually 3). Thus, when an initial test dose suggests that a patient is very sensitive to the sedating effects of the anesthetic agents, consideration can be given to using 1 or 2 increments of the initial bolus rather than all 3. An example of an effective test dose strategy is the slow manual administration of 1 to 2 mL of propofol (or a propofol-remifentanil mixture) immediately after administration of the preinduction dose of midazolam. The rapidity and extent of the patient's response indicate the number of bolus increments that is appropriate for induction.

As mentioned earlier, when the pump is started, its settings must be confirmed to ensure that settings from the previous patient are not inadvertently applied to the current one. Toggling through the confirmation requires less than 10 seconds and helps ensure that the patient is not inadvertently receiving an inappropriate dose. Historically, infusion pumps were too large and cumbersome for most relatively small OMS operatories to accommodate. However, the new digital infusion pumps are small and can be easily attached to an arm on the operating chair or table (Fig. 15). Thus, there is no need for a separate IV stand for mounting the pump.

Once the initial setting is established, intraoperative adjustments are infrequently required. If the face of the pump is covered with a layer of clear sterile autoclave packaging, the surgeon can quickly make pump adjustments during the procedure without having anyone to break scrub, as shown in Fig. 16. It is usually best to establish a foundation level for pump settings. This is the relatively low level at which the average patient responds to the sedating action of the administered agent. Then, if a patient seems to acquire a larger dose, the pump settings can be increased. When the baseline level of the pump setting is set in this manner, it is unlikely that the patient receives an overdose of medication.

An infusion pump not only allows for providing a constant infusion for propofol, it also opens the door to pump-delivered combinations of medications. The importance of the parameter of context-sensitive half-time in evaluating anesthetic medications, especially in regard to discharge considerations, was discussed earlier,. Because of its esterase biotransformation, remifentanil has a low, flat plot of context-sensitive half-time (see Fig. 10). It has been used successfully with propofol in a combined anesthetic for pump delivery. The synergistic effects tend to provide a smooth anesthetic, but one must be mindful of the combined respiratory depressant properties of the combination. Consequently, the senior author prefers to use a ratio of 50 µg of remifentanil to 200 mg of propofol. The complete technique using the propofol/remifentanil combination is as follows:

1. Oral premedication with clonidine, 0.1 to 0.2 mg by mouth
2. Preinduction medications
   a. Midazolam 0.025 mg/kg (approximately 2.0 mg for the average teenager or young adult)
   b. Propofol 1 to 2 mL IV of the combined propofol/remifentanil mixture described earlier (50 µg of remifentanil to 200 mg of propofol) as a test dose; the test dose helps to gauge patient response to the propofol/remifentanil mixture

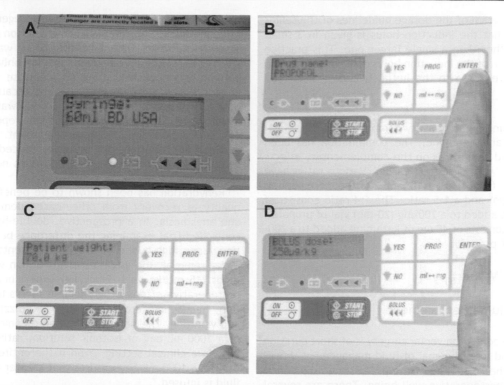

Fig. 14 (*A–D*) Operation of the Aitecs Pro 12S infusion pump: (*A*) The pump senses the type of syringe. (*B*) Programming propofol for drug delivery. (*C*) Programming the patient's weight. (*D*) programming the bolus increment as one-third of the total induction bolus. (*Courtesy of* Richard C. Robert, DDS, MS, South San Francisco, CA.)

   c. Glycopyrrolate 0.003 mg/kg (0.2–0.3 mg for the average teenager or young adult)
   d. Dexamethasone 8 mg as an antiemetic
   e. Diphenhydramine 12.5 to 25 mg as an antiemetic

3. Induction using the propofol/remifentanil mixture (50 μg of remifentanil/200 mg of propofol) and ketamine
   a. The induction rate for the propofol/remifentanil mixture is 750 μg/kg
   b. Ketamine: a manual bolus equal to half of the number of milligrams of propofol bolus administered
4. Maintenance infusion
   a. 50 to 75 μg/kg/min
   b. If necessary, small increments of ketamine 5 to 10 mg can be administered at 10-minute to 15-minute intervals during the procedure; such incremental boluses are used routinely in younger patients

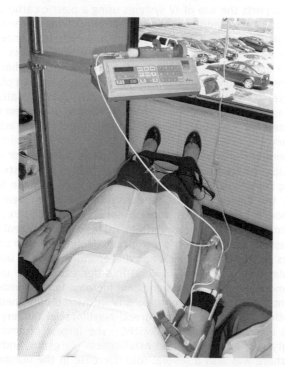

Fig. 15 Mounting of the infusion pump on the light column of the operating chair. This system eliminates the need for a separate IV stand and provides easy access for the operator. (*Courtesy of* Richard C. Robert, DDS, MS, South San Francisco, CA.)

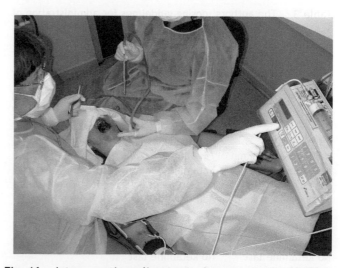

Fig. 16 Intraoperative adjustment of pump settings using sterilization tubing to cover the face of the pump. (*Courtesy of* Richard C. Robert, DDS, MS, South San Francisco, CA.)

5. Table 3 is a diagram of the dosage guidelines of the senior author. Note that the induction bolus is given in 3 small increments rather than a single larger one. This practice enables titration of the induction bolus commensurate with the patient's response to the initial test dose described earlier.

Another intriguing pump delivery combination is an admixture of propofol and ketamine. The combination has been termed Ketofol and capitalizes on the complementary effects of the agents that were described earlier. Various ratios have been used, ranging from 1:1 to 1:10, and 2 of the more popular ones are a 1:4 ratio[8] and a 1:5 ratio. The 1:4 ratio consists of 50 mg of ketamine added to a 200-mg (20-mL) vial of propofol, and the 1:5 ratio consists of 40 mg of ketamine added to a 200-mg (20-mL) vial of propofol.

Perioperative IV therapy

IV Fluids for Volume Replacement

Because office-based dentoalveolar surgery is of short duration with minimal blood loss, the goal of fluid management should not only include the correction of the preexisting fluid deficit but also improve postoperative well-being. There are several adverse outcomes after general anesthesia in ambulatory surgery, including nausea, vomiting, dizziness, drowsiness, thirst, myalgia, sore throat, and delayed recovery. Among possible contributing factors, including anesthetic technique, surgical procedure, duration of surgery, and fluid status of the patient, fluid status is perhaps least frequently reported with clear guidelines. This section regarding fluid management specifically focuses on the best available evidence for the choice and delivery of IV fluids in outpatient dentoalveolar surgery.

Physiologic replacement of the preexisting fluid deficit secondary to preoperative fasting guidelines can be achieved with 0.45% saline solution or 0.9% saline solution. However, the latter, as an isotonic solution, remains within the intravascular space for a longer period and tends to counteract the vasodilatation secondary to anesthetic agents. In contradistinction, infusion of isotonic glucose solution (eg, 5% glucose) is essentially the equivalent of infusion of water, because the glucose is rapidly metabolized, leaving only water. Thus hypotonic agents such as D5W (5% dextrose in water) do not provide equivalent physiologic benefit because of rapid distribution and equilibration with total body water. Furthermore, hypotonic glucose solutions have been reported to increase CO_2 production and respiratory quotient. Given the short duration of outpatient dentoalveolar procedures, withholding glucose in the perioperative period does not predispose patients to hypoglycemia or ketosis.

Rehydration has been shown to be beneficial in improving quality of recovery from office-based dentoalveolar surgery and anesthesia. In a prospective, double-blind, randomized, controlled trial examining the difference between low-hydration versus high-hydration groups in patients undergoing third molar removal, the group receiving a high volume of isotonic fluids (15 mL/kg vs 1–2 mL/kg) experienced fewer adverse postoperative effects. High volume favors less residual sedation, headaches, drowsiness, fatigue, dizziness, and nausea and vomiting. The practical solution recommended is the use of a 1000-mL bag of isotonic solution, rather than a 250-mL bag. In a clinical setting, even if the entire bag is not used, using the 1000-mL bag ensures that greater volume if isotonic fluid is infused.[9]

IV Catheter Systems

The AAOMS Parameters and Pathways recommend that when patients receive medications for deep sedation, IV access should be maintained throughout the procedure until the patient is no longer at risk for cardiopulmonary depression. Safe anesthetic practice requires a reliable venous route for the administration of drugs, and there is a large body of evidence that supports the use of IV systems using a plastic catheter as opposed to the traditional straight needle or winged needle of the butterfly type. The butterfly or similar designed needles are easily inserted and readily fixed to skin. Nonetheless, they can be easily dislodged, and the dangerous sharp needlepoint is more likely to cause laceration and infiltrations than plastic catheters. Although there is a slight risk of plastic catheter blockage, this can be circumvented by the use of a larger bore catheter, or running an infusion continuously to ensure patency.

There are several factors that can be responsible for complications related to venipuncture and IV fluid administration during anesthesia. Amongst these are the nature of the agent itself, the device used for venipuncture and the presence or absence of a continuous infusion during the procedure. The current AAOMS benchmark data in Tables 1 and 2 reveal that the last decade has seen a significant decrease in the use of agents such as methohexital and diazepam, which can lead to vascular complications, a several-fold decrease in the use of rigid metal needles, and a significant increase in the number of patients who receive a continuous IV infusion during their anesthetics. Data from the Oral and Maxillofacial Surgery National Insurance Company (OMSNIC), the largest professional liability carrier for oral and maxillofacial surgeons, indicate that there was also a several-fold decrease in the number of phlebitis and other vascular complications during the first decade of the current century compared with the previous decade (Lew N. Estabrooks, OMSNIC, RRG, personal communication, 2013).

Table 3 The authors' dosing guidelines for administration of a propofol-remifentanil infusion with low-dose ketamine, as described in the text

Teens/Adults	Pediatric	Seniors >65 y
Induction bolus: 250 µg/kg × 2–3	Induction bolus: 330 µg/kg × 3	Induction bolus: 60s→150 µg/kg × 3 70s→150 µg/kg × 2 80s→150 µg/kg × 1
Infusion rate: 50–75 µg/kg/min	Infusion rate: 75–100 µg/kg/min	Infusion rate: 25 µg/kg/min
Ketamine bolus: half propofol bolus	Ketamine bolus: half propofol bolus	Ketamine bolus: not recommended
Additional ketamine as needed 10–15 mg every 10–15 min	Additional ketamine 5–10 mg every 10–15 min	Ketamine bolus: not recommended
No ketamine last 10–15 min	No ketamine last 10–15 min	

Courtesy of Richard C. Robert, DDS, MS, South San Francisco, CA.

Preemptive management of postoperative nausea and vomiting

Historically, postoperative nausea and vomiting (PONV) have been dreaded but common occurrences after IV sedation or general anesthesia. In surveys of postanesthetic outcomes, fear of nausea and vomiting often ranks second only to the fear of death from anesthesia. The marked concern professed by patients has prompted PONV to be characterized as the big little problem in the anesthesia literature. It has also led to a considerable body of research to elucidate the causes and develop management strategies to prevent PONV. In current practice it is common for several antiemetic medications to be administered prophylactically to prevent this highly undesirable outcome.

The main triggers for PONV are general anesthesia with inhalational anesthetics, opioids, and nitrous oxide.[10] A recent systematic review of prospective studies conducted by Apfel and colleagues[11] showed that the most reliable independent predictors of PONV were female gender, history of PONV or motion sickness (MS), nonsmoker, younger age, duration of anesthesia with volatile anesthetics, and postoperative opioids. Apfel and colleagues have also described a simplified risk scoring system to predict PONV, as shown in Fig. 17. The 4 risk factors included in the final simple sum score were female gender, previous history of MS or PONV, nonsmoking, and the use of postoperative opioids. If no risk factor is present, or if there is only 1 risk factor, the incidence of PONV may vary between 10% and 21%, whereas if at least 2 risk factors are present, it may increase to between 39% and 78%.

Spectrum of Receptors

During the last decade and a half, it has become apparent that what has made effective management of PONV so elusive is that there is such a wide variety of receptors that are involved in the altered physiology responsible for nausea and vomiting. The brainstem vomiting center, as shown in Fig. 18, orchestrates the complex act of vomiting. High concentrations of the following receptors are present in the vomiting center:

histamine (H_1), muscarinic (M_1), serotonin (5-HT_3), and neurokinin 1 (NK_1). In addition, the chemoreceptor trigger zone, which is accessible to emetogenic stimuli in the blood or cerebrospinal fluid, is rich in dopamine (D_2) and opioid receptors. A diverse group of antiemetic drugs are available that have affinity for various aforementioned receptors, as shown in Table 4. Most of the available drugs fall within 8 different categories. All of these drugs with the exception of dexamethasone act as antagonists at the corresponding receptor sites. Because so many receptor sites are involved, a single drug is often ineffective in prevention. Thus, in current anesthesia practice, a multimodal approach is used, with the administration of several medications, which exert their effects at different receptor sites.

In the past, anesthetic agents were looked on as the stimuli that induced the nausea and vomiting associated with anesthesia. However, the advent of propofol has altered that concept. Rather than causing nausea and vomiting, propofol has excellent antiemetic properties and can be used with a benzodiazepine for deep sedation in patients with a strong history of PONV.[10] Propofol can even be used independently as an antiemetic rather than just an anesthetic agent. Its antiemetic properties can be attributed to its interactions with D_2 and 5-HT_3 receptors.

During the last decade, a new class of antiemetic agents, the 5-HT_3 antagonists, have revolutionized the medical management of nausea and vomiting. Originally introduced as agents to control the nausea and vomiting that accompany chemotherapy of cancer, these agents soon found a place in the armamentarium of anesthesiologists to manage PONV. Their popularity has been based on both unparalleled efficacy and their favorable side effect profile. The prototypical drug in this group is ondansetron, and it has become the most widely used of the 5-HT_3 antagonists. However, pharmacologic research continued and led to the introduction of palonosetron, a novel 5-HT_3 receptor antagonist with a greater binding affinity and longer half-life than the original 5-HT_3 antagonists. In a randomized, double-blind study published by Kovac and colleagues, a single 0.075-mg IV dose of palonosetron effectively reduced the severity of nausea and delayed the time to emesis and treatment failure in the inpatient surgical setting.

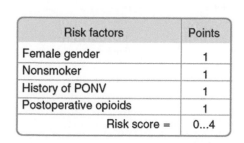

Risk factors	Points
Female gender	1
Nonsmoker	1
History of PONV	1
Postoperative opioids	1
Risk score =	0...4

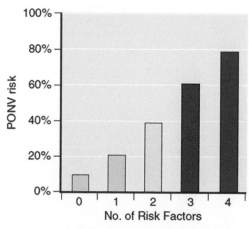

Fig. 17 Simplified risk score for predicting PONV as described by Apfel and colleagues. On the right is a bar chart showing the percentage of PONV risk corresponding to the number of risk factors. (*From* Miller RD. Miller's anesthesia. 7th edition. Philadelphia: Churchill Livingstone/Elsevier; 2010. p. 3084, I-89, with permission; and Apfel CC, Läärä E, Koivuranta M, et al. A simplified risk score for predicting postoperative nausea and vomiting: conclusions from cross-validations between 2 centers. Anesthesiology 1999;91(3):2739; with permission.)

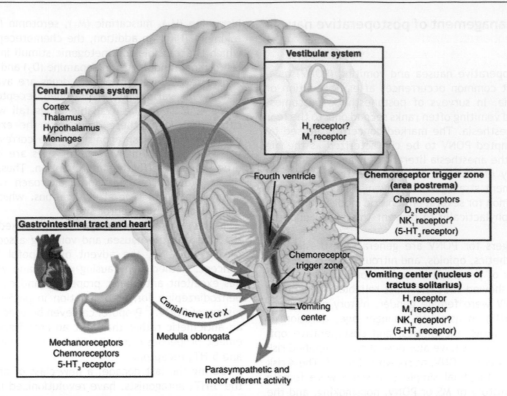

Fig. 18 The CNS centers and receptors for control of emesis and vomiting. (*From* Katzung BG, Masters SB, Trevor AJ. Basic & clinical Q11Q17 pharmacology. 12th edition. McGraw-Hill; 2012. *Adapted from* Krakauer EL, Zhu AX, Bounds BC, et al. Case records of the Massachusetts General Hospital. Weekly clinicopathological exercises. Case 6-2005. A 58-year-old man with esophageal cancer and nausea, vomiting, and intractable hiccups. N Engl J Med 2005;352(8):817–25; with permission.)

Although it is apparent that palonosetron will become popular as an effective antiemetic in a clinical setting, its high cost will probably prevent it from doing so until the original patent expires and a generic form becomes available.

Dexamethasone is a long-acting glucocorticoid with a 36-hour to 54-hour duration of action that has been commonly used in OMS to counteract postoperative edema. However, it is been found that the agent is also efficacious for the prevention

Table 4 Major categories of antiemetic drugs available and their affinity for various receptors. All of these drugs except dexamethasone act as antagonists of the corresponding receptors

Pharmacologic Group	Dopamine (D$_2$)	Muscarinic (M$_1$)	Histamine (H$_1$)	Serotonin (5-HT$_3$)	Neurokinin 1 (NK$_1$)
Anticholinergics					
Scopolamine	+	++++	+	−	−
Antihistamines					
Diphenhydramine	+	++	++++	−	−
Hydroxyzine	+	++	++++	−	−
Promethazine	++	++	++++	−	−
Antiserotonins					
Ondansetron	−	−	−	++++	−
Palonosteron	−	−	−	++++	−
Benzamides					
Metoclopramide	+++	−	−	++	
Butyrophenones					
Droperidol	++++	−	+	+	−
Haloperidol	++++	−	+	−	−
Phenothiazines					
Chlorpromazine	++++	++	++++	+	−
Prochlorperazine	++++	++	++	+	−
Steroids					
Dexamethasone	−	−	−	−	−
Antineurokinins					
Aprepitant	−	−	−	−	++++
Fosaprepitant	−	−	−	−	++++

Adapted from Scuderi PE. Pharmacology of antiemetics. Int Anesthesiol Clin 2003;41(4):42; with permission.

of nausea and vomiting that occurs in the several days after the procedure. The antiemetic mechanism of dexamethasone is not fully understood, but it may involve central inhibition of prostaglandin synthesis, antiinflammatory action, and reduction of 5-HT_3 excretion from the gastrointestinal tract. In addition, it may decrease 5-HT_3 turnover in the CNS or change the permeability of the blood-cerebrospinal fluid barrier to serum proteins.[12] The addition of intraoperative dexamethasone 8 mg to IV ondansetron 4 mg in combination with ondansetron oral dissolving tablets 8 mg dosed immediately before discharge and on postoperative days 1 and 2 significantly reduced the incidence of postdischarge nausea and vomiting and its negative impact on quality of life between the eighth and 120th hours after anesthesia.[12]

In 2001, the US Food and Drug Administration (FDA) issued a black-box warning for droperidol because of a potentially life-threatening side effect. In high doses, droperidol is known to cause QT interval prolongation, which has been associated with cardiac arrhythmias, torsades de pointes, ventricular tachycardia, and cardiac arrest. As an alternative, haloperidol, a butyrophenone congener of droperidol, has been shown to be effective in both preventing and treating PONV. It can be administered both intramuscularly and IV.

Another important antiemetic-related side effect is caused by the parenterally administered promethazine. In 2009, the FDA required a boxed warning for promethazine injection to better communicate the risk of severe tissue injury associated with the injectable form of this drug.[10] Promethazine should neither be administered into an artery nor administered under the skin because of the risk of severe tissue injury, including gangrene. There is also a risk that the drug can leach out from the vein during IV administration and cause severe damage to the surrounding tissue. This situation is more likely to occur when it is administered as an undiluted IV bolus. The preferred parenteral route of administration is injecting the drug intramuscularly.

Substance P or NK_1 receptor antagonists are a new class of antiemetics. They are significantly more efficacious against postoperative vomiting (but not nausea) than other antiemetics. The prototypic drug in this class is aprepitant. Fosprepitant is a prodrug of aprepitant and is administered IV and is approved only for chemotherapy-induced nausea and vomiting. The combination of aprepitant 40 mg and dexamethasone 10 mg was more effective than ondansetron 4 mg and dexamethasone 10 mg for prophylaxis against postoperative vomiting in adult patients undergoing craniotomy under general anesthesia. However, there was no difference in the incidence or severity of nausea.[12]

The multimodal approach for prophylaxis for PONV
As mentioned earlier, because of the complex physiology of nausea and vomiting no current single antiemetic is completely effective in all patients. However, because of the involvement of multiple receptors involved, combination or multimodal therapy has shown enhanced effectiveness. The most frequently studied combinations include ondansetron with droperidol, dexamethasone, or metoclopramide. Early studies[11] have shown that both ondansetron plus dexamethasone and ondansetron plus droperidol were more efficacious than any of the agents used alone. More recent studies have confirmed that a combination of 5-HT_3 antagonist with either droperidol or dexamethasone is superior in efficacy to monotherapy. In 1 recent study, it was shown that a combination of triple antiemetic prophylaxis consisting of droperidol 0.625 mg and

dexamethasone 10 mg administered IV after induction plus ondansetron 1 mg given IV at emergence led to 0% incidence of vomiting in the postanesthesia care unit versus 7% and 22% in the ondansetron monotherapy and placebo groups, respectively. Because histamine receptors are also involved in mediating nausea/vomiting, diphenhydramine can also be used as part of the multiple-agent approach for prevention of PONV.

Over the last couple of years, many oral and maxillofacial surgeons have opted to use more ketamine because of the shortage of propofol. Although ketamine is an excellent drug in small amounts, when it is used as the primary IV anesthetic, the risk of PONV increases. In these cases, multimodal therapy for PONV prevention is even more important. We have found that routine use of the following antiemetic agents has essentially eliminated the incidence of PONV in our patient population: (1) use of propofol when it is available as a primary anesthetic to capitalize on its potent antiemetic properties (5-HT_3, D_2); (2) ondansetron 6 mg IV at the beginning of the case if ketamine is the primary anesthetic, or at the end if propofol is the primary anesthetic (5-HT_3); (3) diphenhydramine 25 mg IV along with the preinduction medications (muscarinic receptors). (4) dexamethasone 8 mg IV in all patients without contraindications to its use and who receive an IV anesthetic, regardless of whether the patient needs the corticosteroid to decrease postoperative edema. (5) metoclopramide 10 mg IV in particularly high-risk patients (D_2). With this low dose, extrapyramidal side effects are infrequent and can be countered with diphenhydramine. An alternative D_2 receptor antagonist is low-dose haloperidol 2 mg IV.

Management of the patient with a high-risk airway in office-based anesthesia

Obesity

Although there are several factors that may affect the difficulty of airway maintenance during anesthesia, obesity is frequently the pivotal predisposing factor for many of them. Obesity is a metabolic disease in which adipose tissue represents a proportion of body mass tissue greater than normal, and its increased prevalence has been one of the most important epidemiologic phenomena in the last century. Most applicable to oral and maxillofacial surgeons in an outpatient setting is recognition of the obese patient with consideration of comorbidities such as OSA and gastroesophageal reflux disease (GERD). The following is a discussion concerning the management of comorbidities in the setting of airway assessment, patient positioning, and postoperative pain control.

Clinically, obesity is frequently defined by the following 3 criteria: (1) height/weight index, (2) ratio of actual and ideal weight, and (3) body mass index (BMI, calculated as weight in kilograms divided by the square of height in meters). The value of BMI lies in simple computation and its known correlation with the risk of morbidity and mortality. The calculation is as follows: BMI = (wt. in kg ÷ ht. in m^2) or BMI = (wt. in lbs. ÷ ht. in inches) × 703.

Typically, overweight is defined as a BMI (Fig. 19) between 25 and 30 kg/m^2, obese defined as between 30 to 40 kg/m^2, and morbidly obese defined as greater than 40 kg/m^2 (or 35 kg/m^2 with comorbidities).[13] Data from the National Center for Health Statistics, Centers for Disease Control and Prevention for 2009 to 2010 indicated a prevalence of obesity of 35% to 36% in the US population. The current AAOMS benchmark study

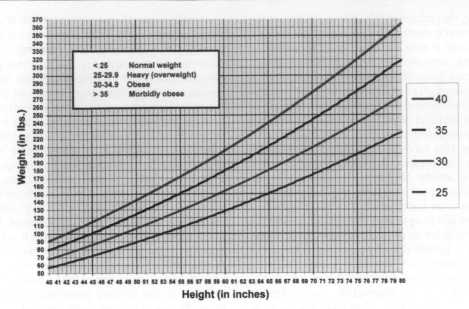

Fig. 19 Graphic BMI calculator for rapid determination of the patient's BMI based on the patient's weight in pounds and height in inches. (*Courtesy of* Richard C. Robert, DDS, MS, South San Francisco, CA.)

found that approximately 24% of patients receiving IV anesthesia were obese as defined by a BMI greater than 30 (Table 5). It has been suggested that patients who have a BMI of greater than 35 may not be acceptable candidates for anesthesia in an office setting.[13] A reasonable interpretation of the disparity between the percentage of obese patients in the general population and those receiving anesthesia in OMS is that many obese patients are now being treated in an outpatient surgery center or hospital setting as opposed to the OMS office.

In general, the calculation of dosages of agents for induction of anesthesia should be based on ideal body weight (IBW) rather than total body weight (TBW). IBW can be estimated as follows: adult male IBW (kg) = height (cm) − 100, and adult female IBW (kg) = height (cm) − 105. In a clinical setting, converting this formula to a graphical form lends itself to expedient access (Fig. 20). For maintenance of anesthesia, especially propofol, dosing often needs to be increased and approaches a level more consistent with TBW.

For morbidly obese patients, dosing scalars based on IBW can result in a subtherapeutic dose, whereas TBW can lead to overdose. Lean body weight (LBW) is the most appropriate dosing scalar for most anesthetic agents, including opioids and propofol, in obese patients. LBW is the difference between TBW and fat mass, which increases with TBW but not in a linear fashion. LBW is appropriate because it is significantly

Table 5 Distribution of patients in 2011 to 2012 AAOMS benchmark study by weight category

BMI Category	Frequency	Percent
Normal <24	2440	44.8
Heavy 25–29	1701	31.2
Obese 30–39	1095	20.1
Morbidly obese ≥40	208	3.8
Total	5444	100

Courtesy of Martin L. Gonzalez, MS, Senior Research Associate, American Association of Oral and Maxillofacial Surgeons, Rosemont, IL.

correlated to cardiac output, an important determinant in early distribution kinetics of drugs. Drug clearance also increases proportionately with LBW. As useful as it is, LBW has been limited by the difficulty of its being accurately measured under normal clinical circumstances. James' equation is commonly used, and the graphical form (Fig. 21) is most clinically useful, except at extremes of TBW.[14]

OSA

One of the most serious consequences of obesity is the tendency of the obese to develop OSA. OSA is the most prevalent breathing disorder during sleep. It is characterized by 5 or more episodes of apnea, each lasting more than 10 seconds or causing a decrease in oxyhemoglobin saturation of 4% or more from baseline.[15] Obesity exerts its effects through increasing local compressive forces on the upper airway and by decreasing functional residual capacity (FRC). The net effect is longitudinal traction on the upper airway, particularly when the patient is recumbent (Fig. 22). The factors that predispose to OSA also predispose to obstruction under anesthesia. Factors that pose a risk of narrowing of the airway include increasing age, male gender, menopause, obesity, increased neck circumference, macroglossia, retrognathia, and maxillary constriction (Fig. 23).[16] Cardinal symptoms of OSA include habitual snoring, witnessed apnea, disrupted and unrefreshing sleep, and excessive daytime sleepiness. Signs include obesity, increased neck circumference, mandibular or maxillary hypoplasia, and oropharyngeal crowding (Fig. 24).[16]

Although snoring is a primary symptom of OSA and is almost 100% sensitive for the diagnosis, it has low specificity and positive predictive value when used alone. Although polysomnography (PSG) is the gold standard in the diagnosis of OSA, it is expensive, time-consuming, and requires trained personnel. Thus, it is not practical to perform PSG in all patients suspected of suffering from OSA. Consequently, efforts have been directed at developing practical OSA screening tools. One of these, the STOP-Bang Questionnaire shown in Table 6, has been shown to be particularly helpful in

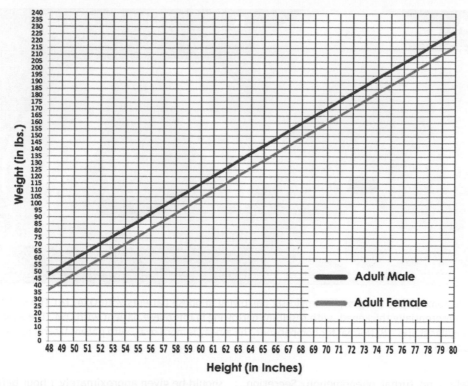

Fig. 20 IBW graphic calculator: quick conversion to IBW based on height and weight. (*Courtesy of* Richard C. Robert, DDS, MS, South San Francisco, CA.)

identification of patients at high risk of OSA.[15] It is composed of 8 simple, straightforward questions, which can be asked rapidly during the preoperative consultation. Using a cutoff of at least 6 positive responses on the STOP-Bang Questionnaire usually identifies patients truly at risk for moderate to severe OSA.[15]

GERD

A second comorbidity linked to obesity that poses a risk for pulmonary complications is GERD. GERD is commonly defined as regurgitation (or heartburn) 2 to 3 times per week. Its incidence in the general population ranges from 8% to 26%, and

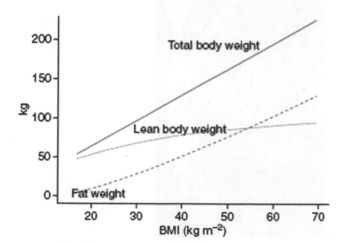

Fig. 21 Relationship of TBW, fat weight, and LBW to BMI in standard height male. (*From* Ingrande J, Lemmens HJ. Dose adjustment of anaesthetics in the morbidly obese. Br J Anaesth 2010;105 (Suppl 1):17; with permission.)

its prevalence is further increased in the obese population. Anesthesia-related aspiration can result in severe aspiration pneumonitis or development of adult respiratory distress syndrome. Although the incidence of perioperative gastrointestinal and pulmonary complications in the routine surgical population is low, there is a changing population demographic with more surgical procedures performed in the elderly. This patient population is likely to have a greater number of preexisting comorbidities, which often include regurgitation and aspiration.

Although the American Society of Anesthesiologists does not recommend the routine administration of acid suppressants to all preoperative patients, it does believe that their use is appropriate for the prevention of morbidity in patients who are considered at risk for aspiration (Box 1). Over the last decade and a half, there has been a shift in the medical management of gastric acid diseases from H_2 receptor antagonists to proton pump inhibitors (PPIs). The PPIs are the most potent and reliable acid suppressants available, and offer the versatility of IV administration. They can also be effective in the management of excessive gastric acid production in the perioperative period. Although in general, they have few side effects and drug interactions, omeprazole has been reported to inhibit diazepam, phenytoin, and warfarin metabolism, whereas lansoprazole increase the metabolism of theophylline. No significant drug interactions have been reported with pantoprazole.

Overall, PPIs have been more effective agents in dealing with acid-related diseases than their predecessors, the H_2 receptor antagonists. However, even with twice-daily dosing, many patients develop acid breakthrough. This finding is mirrored in a recent meta-analysis comparing the efficacy of PPIs and H_2 receptor antagonists to decrease the risk of aspiration during anesthesia. The study found that when both drugs were given by mouth as a single dose before surgery, H_2 receptor antagonists were more effective than PPIs.[17] Gastric

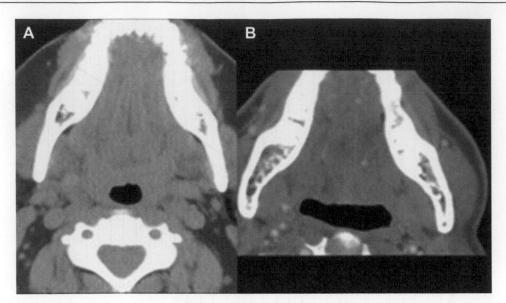

Fig. 22 Axial computed tomography images of retroglossal narrowing in obese patients with OSA. (*A*) The soft tissues around the retroglossal airway are circumferentially thickened, with resultant narrowing in this obese patient with OSA. The airway is round rather than the normal oval or rectangular shape. (*B*) Normal for comparison. The airway is more oval, with patent lateral recesses. (*Courtesy of* David Solsberg, MD, Englewood, CO.)

acid secretion is largely a nocturnal phenomenon. Secretion shows a circadian pattern, in which peak concentration usually occurs at 1 to 2 AM. Therefore, for most patients, a single dose of 300 mg of ranitidine on the evening before surgery is an efficacious approach. The exception is patients who have been on long-term H₂ antagonist therapy. These patients tend to develop tolerance, which usually results in suboptimal gastric acid suppression. In cases such as these, the use of a PPI (eg, esomeprazole 40 mg by mouth) is appropriate. To ensure that the peak serum concentration of the PPI coincides with the maximal activation of proton pump secretion, the medication

should be given approximately 1 hour before the evening meal on the night before surgery.

Positioning and Airway Evaluation of the Obese Patient with the High-Risk Airway

Obese patients have low compliance of the respiratory system and high resistance because of reduced lung volume and expiratory flow limitation, which is accentuated in the supine position. The supine position, anesthesia, and narcotic medications all decrease the FRC. This situation makes airway

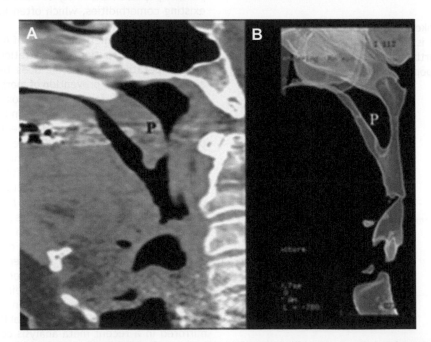

Fig. 23 Sagittal images of a patient with retroglossal narrowing and severe OSA. (*A*) Sagittal reformat view shows the posterior displacement of the enlarged tongue. The palate (P) is also long and thickened, contributing to narrowing of the airway. (*B*) A volume-rendered air-containing structure view shows the marked narrowing of the retroglossal airway even while the patient was awake. (*Courtesy of* David Solsberg, MD, Englewood, CO.)

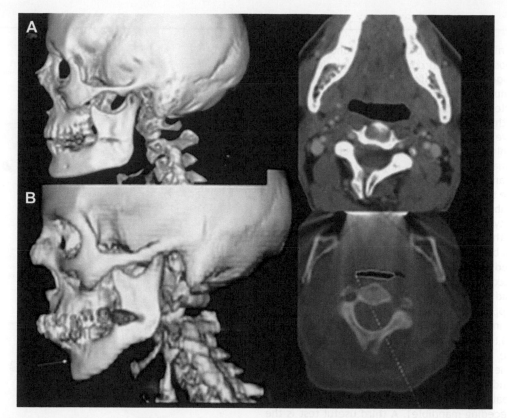

Fig. 24 Patient with small mandible, compared with normal. (*A*) Normal bone three-dimensional volume-rendering image on left with axial image through the retroglossal airway on left. Note that the mandibular size is proportionate to the maxilla and orbits. (*B*) This woman had a thin body habitus but has severe OSA. Note the hypoplastic and receding mandible (*arrow*) and markedly narrowed retroglossal airway on the axial image. (*Courtesy of* David Solsberg, MD, Englewood, CO.)

Table 6 The STOP-Bang questionnaire as described in the text

1. Snoring	
Do you snore loudly (louder than talking or loud enough to be heard through closed doors)?	
Yes	No
2. Tired	
Do you often feel tired, fatigued, or sleepy during daytime?	
Yes	No
3. Observed	
Has anyone observed you stop breathing during your sleep?	
Yes	No
4. Blood pressure	
Do you have or are you being treated for high blood pressure?	
Yes	No
5. BMI	
BMI more than 35 kg/m^2?	
Yes	No
6. Age	
Age older than 50 y?	
Yes	No
7. Neck circumference	
Neck circumference greater than 40 cm?	
Yes	No
8. Gender	
Gender male?	
Yes	No

High risk of OSA: answering yes to 3 or more items.
Low risk of OSA: answering yes to less than 3 items.

From Chung F, Yegneswaran B, Liao P, et al. STOP questionnaire: a tool to screen patients for obstructive sleep apnea. Anesthesiology 2008;108(5):821; with permission.

Box 1. Risk factors for pulmonary aspiration

American Society of Anesthesiologists physical status III or IV
Surgery outside regular working hours[a]
Emergency surgery[a]
Obesity, ascites, large abdominal mass
Gastritis, history of ulcers
Autonomic neuropathy (familial, acquired)
Muscular disorders
Long-lasting general anesthetics
Vocal cord paralysis
Diabetes mellitus
Electrolyte, metabolic imbalance
Insufficient anesthetic depth
Airway difficulty
Preexisting GERD
Esophageal and upper abdominal surgery
Increased intracranial pressure
Degenerative neuropathies
Opioids, methylxanthines, β-agonists
Reduced level of consciousness
Laryngeal malfunction or spasm
Collagen vascular disease
Renal, pelvic, bladder, or uterine distention

[a] Increases risk by 5-fold to 6-fold.

From Atlee JL. Complications in anesthesia. 2nd edition. Philadelphia: Elsevier/Saunders; 2007. p. xxxvi, 994; with permission.

assessment, recognition of comorbidities (OSA and GERD), and familiarity with positioning and compromised airway maneuvers critically important. The safest positioning of obese patients is in a semiupright position during surgery. Care must also be taken in selecting a blood pressure cuff that has a width greater than one-third the circumference of the arm.

For preoperative airway assessment, the Mallampati classification is commonly used, although it is characterized by low sensitivity, reasonable specificity (Fig. 25), low positive predictive value, and significant false-positive results. Consequently, as a single screening tool for the difficult airway it has limitations. A combination of several screening tools is more effective than any one used separately. A second useful screening test for the high-risk airway is the upper lip bite test (ULBT), which has been shown to have greater specificity and accuracy compared with the Mallampati classification.[18] The ULBT takes into account both jaw architecture and tooth position (Fig. 26), and is divided into 3 classes: (1) lower incisors biting into the upper lip above the level of the vermillion border, (2) lower incisors biting into the upper lip within the vermillion; and (3) lower incisors fail to bite the upper lip. The hypothesis for the improved specificity and accuracy results from its simultaneous assessment of jaw subluxation and presence of protruding teeth, 2 of the 5 risk factors that predict difficult intubation (others include weight, head and neck movement, and receding mandible). A third useful test is the

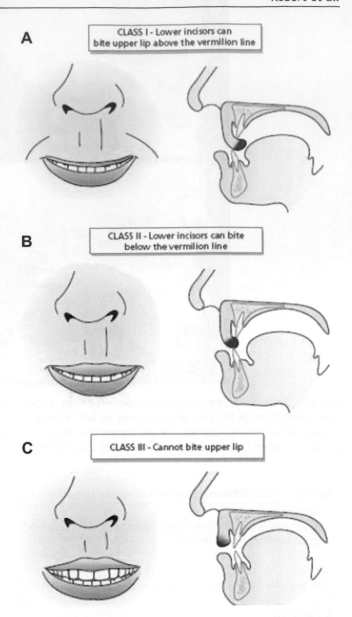

Fig. 26 The ULBT, as described in the text. (*From* Khan Z, Kashif A, Ebrahimkhani E. A comparison of the upper lip bite test. Anesth Analg 2003:96:595—9; with permission.)

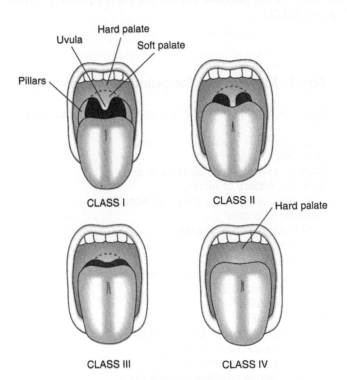

Class I: Full visibility of tonsils, uvula and soft palate.
Class II: Visibility of hard and soft palate, upper portion of tonsils and uvula.
Class III: Soft and hard palate and base of the uvula are visible.
Class IV: Only hard palate visible.

Fig. 25 The Mallampati classification. (*From* Morgan GE, Mikhail MS, Murray MJ. Clinical anesthesiology. 4th ed. New York: Lange Medical Books/McGraw Hill, Medical Pub. Division; 2006; with permission.)

sternomental distance, which is the linear distance between the upper border of the manubrium of the sternum and the bony point of the chin. A measurement of 12.5 cm or less with the head fully extended on the neck and the mouth closed indicates difficult intubation (and presumably difficult airway management during office-based anesthesia).

Airway Adjuncts of Benefit in the Management of the High-Risk Airway

Nasopharyngeal catheter

A nasopharyngeal catheter (trumpet) is a useful airway adjunct for patients with a difficult airway. It can be used in a minimally sedated patient as well as a moderately or deeply sedated patient or patient under general anesthesia. However, there is a caveat in that the catheter must be sufficiently long to pass behind the tongue (Fig. 27). Once the catheter has been placed, a Weider retractor can be used to visualize the oropharynx and ensure that the tip is long enough to extend behind the tongue. If it seems that the regular trumpet configuration airway of appropriate diameter is not of sufficient length, a nasopharyngeal catheter (Teleflex Incorporated, Limerick, PA, USA) with an adjustable sleeve is available, as shown in Fig. 28.

Laryngeal mask airway

The laryngeal mask airway (LMA; [LMA North America, San Diego, CA, USA]) has been used for both emergency airway intervention as well as administration of tube-delivered anesthesia. An LMA consists of a wide-bore tube, the proximal end of which is connected to a breathing circuit and the distal end is fitted to an elliptical cuff that covers the entrance to the larynx and is inflated through a pilot, as shown in Fig. 29. In preparation for insertion, the cuff is deflated and lubricated (Fig. 30). The tube is grasped as if holding a pencil and inserted blindly into the hypopharynx, such that the cuff forms a low-pressure seal around the laryngeal entrance when inflated. LMAs intended for establishment of an emergency airway are relatively stiff and not sufficiently flexible to enable deflection

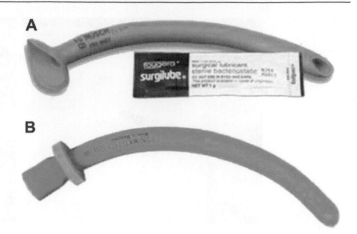

Fig. 28 Configurations of nasopharyngeal airways. (*A*) The conventional trumpet configuration. (*B*) An adjustable-length nasopharyngeal airway.

of the tube out of the surgical field during OMS procedures. However, there is a more flexible armored LMA constructed of a pliable plastic in which is embedded a metal spiral to prevent collapse of the lumen (Fig. 31).

Placement of the LMA is less stimulating than intubation with a endotracheal tube and laryngoscope. A 10% to 20% increase in the induction bolus of propofol normally used for dentoalveolar procedures is usually adequate to allow placement of the LMA. The armored LMA can be moved from side to side within the oral cavity to allow surgical procedures to be performed on the contralateral side. The LMA partially protects the larynx from pharyngeal secretions (but not gastric regurgitation), and it should remain in place until the patient has regained airway reflexes.

Tongue traction suture

A simple airway adjunct that requires no special equipment and ease of application is a tongue traction suture. A double 3-0 chromic or silk suture is placed through the dorsum of the tongue near the midline at the junction of the middle and anterior thirds (Fig. 32). The sutures are secured with a Kelly hemostat, which is placed at the commissure contralateral to the operative site. In most cases, gravitational forces on the hemostat provide traction with the hemostat draped over the commissure. However, light traction can be placed on the hemostat by a surgical assistant if additional traction is necessary. This airway adjuncts has the added advantage of providing control of the tongue during placement of the posterior oral packing and the surgical procedure itself.

Mandibular traction wire

In patients who are retrognathic or have large tongues, just a few millimeters of anterior posturing of the mandible is sufficient to reposition the tongue anteriorly to open an airway occluded by a retro positioned tongue. A 24-gauge wire can be passed between the first and second M teeth to the medial aspect of the mandible. It then passes lingual to the posterior teeth and is finally passed to the buccal again between the first premolar and cuspid. The ends are twisted together with a wire twister, which can be used for translation of the mandibular condyle anteriorly (Fig. 33) during surgery. In addition, this anterior repositioning of the mandible enhances surgical access to the third molar region and the mandibular ramus.

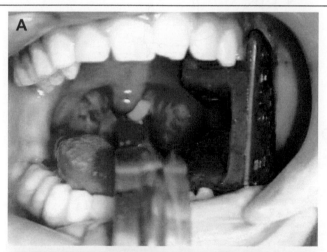

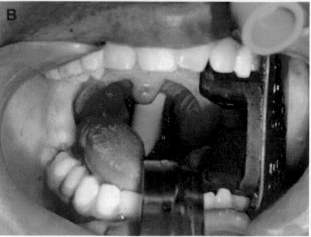

Fig. 27 Confirming appropriate placement of the nasopharyngeal catheter. If the tip of the conventional trumpet catheter does not pass behind the tongue as in (*A*), an adjustable-length catheter can be used to provide adequate length for appropriate tip positioning, as in (*B*).

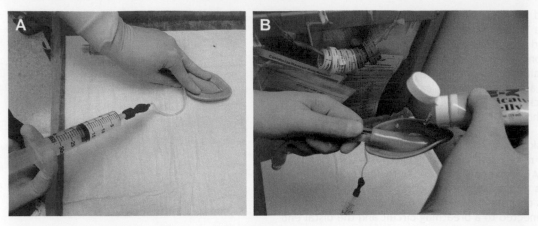

Fig. 29 (A–B) Preparation of the LMA for insertion. (A) The cuff is deflated with a 30-mL syringe such that the rims of the cuff are deflected away from the laryngeal structures. (B) The mask is lubricated liberally with a water-soluble lubricant.

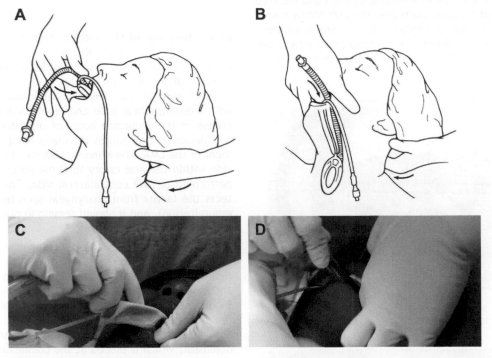

Fig. 30 (A–D) Placement of the LMA. (A) Hand positioning for conventional placement from the head of the table. (B) Passing the index finger of the opposite hand along the tube to ensure proper positioning of the airway over the larynx. (C) Alternative placement of the tube from the patient's side. (D) Side approach: passage of the forefinger of the opposite hand beside the airway tube to ensure proper positioning of the mask over the larynx. (*Courtesy of* Richard C. Robert, DDS, MS, South San Francisco, CA.)

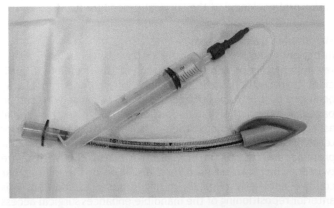

Fig. 31 The armored flexible LMA. (*See text for description.*)

Postoperative Care of the High-Risk Airway Patient

In the high-risk airway patient, postoperative opioids, sedatives, and tranquilizers that reduce the patient's defenses against airway obstruction can lead to serious morbidity and even mortality.[19] OMSNIC closed-claim data show that postoperative opioid pain medication is a leading cause of anesthetic deaths after discharge (Lew N. Estabrooks, OMSNIC, RRG, personal communication, 2013). The anesthesia provider must be acutely aware of the mechanisms of the body in its depressed response to hypoxemia and hypercarbia because of the effects of opioids and sedatives on pharyngeal tone, carotid chemoreceptor function, and brainstem respiratory receptors.[19] There is also the concern of residual effects of anesthetic drugs during the first 24 hours after discharge. The

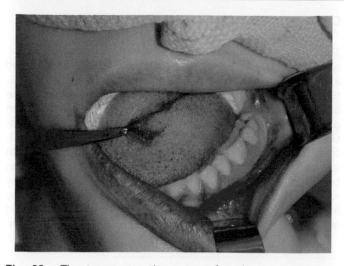

Fig. 32 The tongue traction suture for airway maintenance during office-based anesthesia. (*See text for description.*) (*Courtesy of* Richard C. Robert, DDS, MS, South San Francisco, CA.)

postoperative patient may also have been sleep deprived because of preprocedural anxiety. When sleep-deprived patients achieve real sleep, they can reach deep levels of REM sleep, which leads to muscle relaxation that can precipitate obstruction of the airway.[19]

The combination of appropriate postoperative monitoring and use of nonopioid pain medications is crucial. A reasonable approach is to use 30 mg of ketorolac given IV at the end of procedure followed by 10 mg given orally every 4 to 6 hours during the evening. Narcotics such as Vicodin can be taken during the early day hours when the patient is awake. For the morbidly obese patient, continuous positive airway pressure should be considered. The patient should also remain in a semirecumbent position (30°–45°) during the first 2 to 3 days postoperatively, when postoperative edema is at its maximum.

Methods for monitoring ventilation

Monitoring of the respiratory system during anesthesia has 2 components: the monitoring of ventilation and the monitoring of oxygenation. The AAOMS benchmark data from 2011 to 2012 are

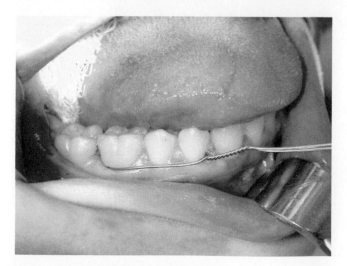

Fig. 33 The mandibular anterior traction wire for airway maintenance during office-based anesthesia. (*See text for description.*) (*Courtesy of* Richard C. Robert, DDS, MS, South San Francisco, CA.)

Table 7 Respiratory monitoring of patients in 2011 to 2012 AAOMS benchmark study

Method	Frequency	Percent
Pulse oximetry	2569	99.7
Monitoring of chest movement	2171	84.2
Precordial/pretracheal stethoscope	1138	44.2
Capnograph	150	5.8
Total	6028	233.9

Courtesy of Martin L. Gonzalez, MS, Senior Research Associate, American Association of Oral and Maxillofacial Surgeons, Rosemont, IL.

tabulated in Table 7. The data indicate that the most frequently used respiratory monitor is the pulse oximeter, which measures oxygen saturation as an indirect indication of oxygenation. The most frequently used method of monitoring ventilation is the least exact (ie, chest movement). Although more definitive methods of monitoring ventilation are available, they are less frequently used. Auscultation with a pretracheal/precordial stethoscope is used in only 44.2% of cases and capnography in only 5.8%, yet closed-claims data from OMSNIC indicate that the most frequent reason for transfer of an OMS patient under anesthesia to an emergency room is respiratory distress (Lew N. Estabrooks, OMSNIC, RRG, personal communication, 2013). Thus, proper preoperative workup, intraoperative airway management, and respiratory status monitoring are critical.

Although pulse oximetry is the most frequently used method of respiratory monitoring, it has a significant limitation in that it lacks real-time responsiveness to significant respiratory events such as airway obstruction or respiratory depression. This situation is best shown by the nature of the oxyhemoglobin dissociation curve (Fig. 34).[20] The curve has a sigmoid

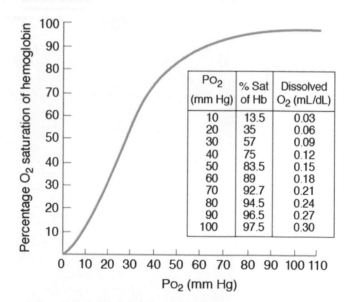

Fig. 34 The oxyhemoglobin dissociation curve. Note that a large decrease in Pao$_2$ does not produce a significant decrease in Sao$_2$ until the steeper portion of the curve is encountered at a Pao$_2$ of 70 mm Hg, which corresponds to Sao$_2$ of 92.7%. Therefore, pulse oximetry may not detect a hypoxemic event until well after it has occurred. (*From* Barrett KE, Barman SM, Boitano S, et al. Ganong's review of medical physiology. New York, NY: McGraw-Hill; 2012; with permission.)

configuration such that a large decrease in partial pressure of oxygen (Pa_{O_2}) does not produce a significant decrease in oxygen saturation (Sa_{O_2}) until the steeper portion of the oxygen hemoglobin dissociation curve is encountered at a Pa_{O_2} of approximately 60 to 70 mm Hg. This finding is particularly important in patients receiving supplemental oxygen. For example, a decrease in Pa_{O_2} in a patient from 130 to 65 mm Hg is required before a significant decrease in Sa_{O_2} is detected. Therefore, the pulse oximeter may not detect a hypoxemic event until well after it has occurred. In a study by Choi and colleagues,[21] the desaturation response time of oxygen saturation to 95% after apnea caused by induction of anesthesia without preoxygenation was 94 seconds. A delay of more than a minute and a half in the face of a significant airway obstruction or respiratory depression could be catastrophic.

Capnography

The shortcomings of pulse oximetry in respiratory monitoring were appreciated early on, and research efforts were directed at the development of a parameter that would provide a real-time assessment. The result was capnography, which is the noninvasive measurement of the partial pressure of carbon dioxide (CO_2) from the airway during inspiration and expiration. Unlike pulse oximetry, it does provide real-time sensitivity to early changes in ventilation and is reliable even in low-perfusion states. Initially, capnographic equipment was bulky and expensive, which limited its use to hospital operating rooms. The more recent introduction of infrared spectroscopy has led to the development of capnographs that can be used outside the operating rooms.[22] In October 2010, in recognition

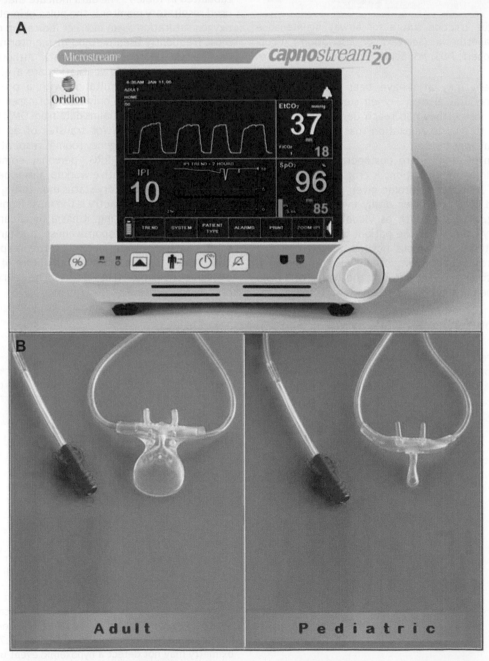

Fig. 35 Capnography equipment. (*A*) A typical sidestream capnography unit. (*B*) Adult and pediatric CO_2 sampling devices used with the capnography unit shown. These devices are also used for oxygen delivery; oxygen delivery tubing is not shown here. Nasal prongs sample CO_2 in nose breathers and the oral scoop samples CO_2 in mouth breathers. The orange port connects the sample tubing to the capnography unit.

of the importance of definitive respiratory monitoring for sedation as well as general anesthesia, the American Society of Anesthesiologists published a new standard (with an effective date of July 1, 2011) calling for the use of capnography during moderate or deep sedation. A mandate from the AAOMS Board of Trustees followed, with the establishment of a similar requirement for anesthesia in OMS, which will take effect on January 1, 2014. The 2012 Parameters of Care: Clinical Practice Guidelines for Oral and Maxillofacial Surgery were revised and now require capnographic monitoring during moderate sedation, deep sedation, and general anesthesia. Capnographic monitoring of sedated patients consists of a sidestream capnograph and a CO_2 sampling device along with the sample tubing that connects it to the capnograph (Fig. 35).

Capnographs

Infrared spectroscopy-based capnographs have 2 configurations: mainstream (flow through) or sidestream. They both rely on a beam of filtered infrared radiation that is passed through the exhaled air and sensed by a photodetector (Fig. 36).[23] CO_2 absorbs light at a specific wavelength of 4.26 μm. Therefore, the amount of radiation absorbed can be measured and used to calculate the concentration of CO_2.

Mainstream capnographs measure CO_2 passing through a photodetector placed in the breathing circuit. They are designed for use in closed circuits such as in intubated patients. The sensing chamber is large and heavy and is heated to remove water vapor. Consequently, the mainstream configuration capnograph is not practical for monitoring in the OMS

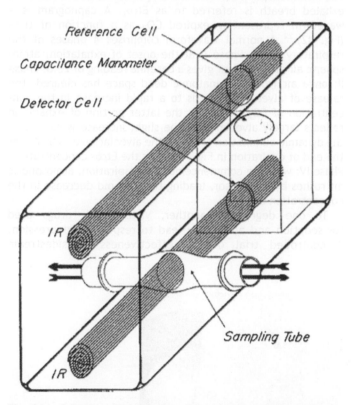

Fig. 36 Schema of pickup box of rapid infrared CO_2 analyzer. Gas flowing through sampling tube traverses 1 infrared path, causing pressure difference between CO_2-filled detector and reference cells. (*From* Jaffe MB. Infrared measurement of carbon dioxide in the human breath: "breathe-through" devices from Tyndall to the present day. Anesth Analg 2008;107(3):894; with permission.)

office. Sidestream capnographs continuously aspirate gas from the breathing circuit through small-caliber tubing to the sensor within the monitor. They can be used in an open anesthesia system such as that used in contemporary office-based OMS practices.

High aspiration rates and sample tubing with low dead space increase sensitivity and decrease lag time. However, sidestream units are prone to water precipitation in the aspiration tube and sampling cell, which can cause obstruction of the sampling line and result in erroneous readings. Fig. 37 shows tracings obtained during mechanical ventilation of an anesthetized patient. The sidestream capnogram lags the mainstream capnogram by the transport time of gas in the capillary connecting the sampling port to the gas analyzer, and the tracing is dampened. Fig. 38 shows capnograms from sidestream capnographs monitoring patients with an open circuit (nasal cannula) and a semiclosed circuit (LMA). Compared with the capnogram associated with a semiclosed circuit, the capnogram associated with an open circuit lacks sharpness and quantitative reliability in the measurement of the end-tidal CO_2 (Etco$_2$) concentration.

CO_2 sampling devices for capnography

In nonintubated patients receiving supplemental oxygen, the insufflated oxygen has the potential to dilute the sampled gases, leading to a large difference between Etco$_2$ and partial pressure of arterial CO_2 (Paco$_2$). Bowe and colleagues modified a nasal cannula by obstructing O_2 flow into 1 prong, thereby permitting O_2 insufflation into 1 nostril while sampling gases from the other nostril. The difference between Paco$_2$ and Etco$_2$ using this device was similar (2.09 + 2.18 mm Hg) to that obtained from the same patients after intubation and mechanical ventilation (2.87 + 2.82 mm Hg). This type of modified nasal cannula (Fig. 39) and other types as shown in Fig. 35 are commercially available for use with capnography in the sedated patient.

For many oral and maxillofacial surgeons, nitrous oxide and oxygen are an integral part of their anesthetic technique. Thus, for those surgeons, any CO_2 sampling device must be compatible with their existing N_2O/O_2 delivery system. Small bore sampling devices have been developed with sampling

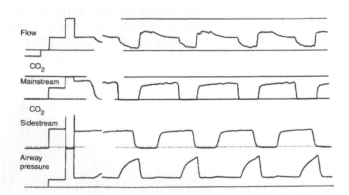

Fig. 37 Tracings from a patient during controlled ventilation. (*From top to bottom*) Flow, mainstream capnogram, sidestream capnogram, and airway pressure. The sidestream capnogram lags behind because the gas has to be carried via a capillary from the patient to the analyzer. This situation also leads to dampening of the waveform. (Gravenstein JS. Clinical Perspectives (Ch. 1) Capnography. 2nd edition. New York: Cambridge University Press; 2011. xiv, 474, p. 2.)

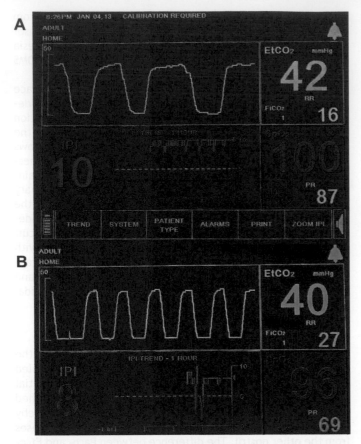

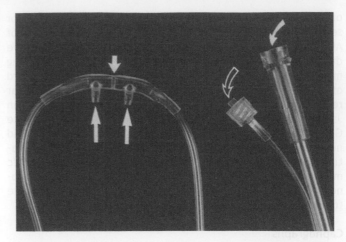

Fig. 39 The 2-prong nasal cannula: one prong supplies O_2 via 1 naris and the other prong samples exhaled gases from the other naris. A septum (*solid short arrow*) separates the 2 prongs (*long solid arrows*) so that there is no gas mixing between the delivery and sampling prongs. The O_2 is supplied via a standard connection (*curved solid arrow*). The connection to capnographic tubing is also shown (*curved hollow arrow*). (*From* Roth JV, Barth LJ, Womack LH, et al. Evaluation of 2 commercially available carbon dioxide sampling nasal cannulae. J Clin Monit 1994;10(4):239; with permission.)

Fig. 38 (*A*) A sidestream capnograph screen monitoring a sedated patient (open circuit) showing normal breathing pattern. CO_2 is sampled using a nasal cannula. (*B*) A sidestream capnograph screen monitoring a general anesthesia patient with an LMA (semiclosed circuit) showing normal breathing pattern. (*Courtesy of* OMS Clinic San Francisco General Hospital, San Francisco, CA; with permission.)

Capnogram interpretation

The maximum partial pressure of CO_2 obtained at the end of an exhaled breath is referred to as $Etco_2$. A capnogram is a waveform representing expired CO_2 as a function of time (Fig. 42).[22] A normal waveform comprises 4 phases of the respiratory cycle. Phase I: at the onset of exhalation, atmospheric air at the sensor gives a baseline reading of zero. Phase II: once air from the anatomic dead space has cleared, the release of alveolar air leads to a rapid increase in the concentration of CO_2. Phase III: the latter portion of exhalation reflects largely alveolar gas. The slight increase is caused by the dynamic elimination of CO_2 at the alveolar level. The dot at the end of expiration in Fig. 42 marks the $Etco_2$ concentration. Phase IV: with the commencement of inspiration, atmospheric air rushes by the sensor, leading to the rapid decrease in the concentration of CO_2.

To one degree or another, virtually all drugs used for sedation and anesthesia lead to respiratory depression. A controlled trial of the effectiveness of sidestream

prongs (Salter Labs, Arvin, CA, USA) that are placed within the nares, as shown in Fig. 40. The fine-bore tubing that attaches the sampling device to the capnograph is sufficiently small that it does not significantly disrupt the adaptation of the N_2O/O_2 mask. Another simple technique is placement of the cut end of a microbore sampling tube at the opening of 1 of the nares (Criticare, Waukesha, WI), as shown in Fig. 41.

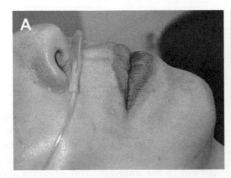

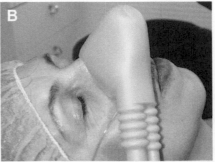

Fig. 40 (*A, B*) CO_2 sampler for use with nitrous oxide oxygen mask. (*A*) The small prongs of the device are placed within the nares. (*B*) The conventional nitrous oxide oxygen mask is placed over the sampling device within the nares. (*Courtesy of* Richard C. Robert, DDS, MS, South San Francisco, CA.)

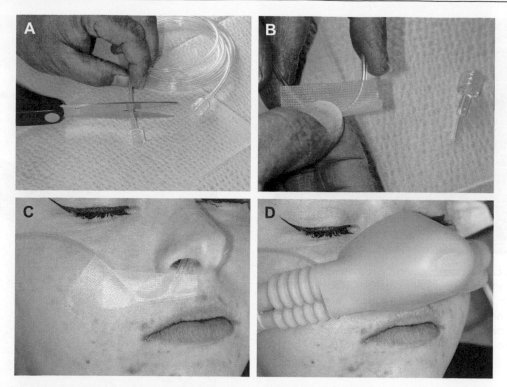

Fig. 41 (*A*) One end of the double-ended Luer-Lock sampling connector is sectioned off with scissors. (*B*) The cut end is bent into a 90°–120° curvature and taped as shown. (*C*) The end of the fine-bore connector tubing is placed at the opening of 1 of the nares and secured to the patient's cheek with tape. (*D*) The fine-bore tubing is sufficiently small that it does not interfere significantly with the seal of the N_2O/O_2 mask. (*Courtesy of* Richard C. Robert, DDS, MS, South San Francisco, CA.)

capnographic monitoring during moderate sedation in the pediatric population published in 2005 showed the early detection of arterial oxygen desaturation caused by alveolar hypoventilation in the presence of supplemental oxygen. In a closed anesthetic system, capnograms provide both qualitative and quantitative information (respiratory rate and $Etco_2$). In an open system, quantitative assessment of $Etco_2$ is less reliable, but the qualitative information provided by the

capnogram morphology and pattern is invaluable. Some of the common capnographic ventilatory patterns that may be encountered in an OMS outpatient practice include interval breathing, hypoventilation, hyperventilation, apnea, laryngospasm, upper airway obstruction, and bronchospasm.[24] Fig. 43 shows the capnographic patterns seen with alveolar hypoventilation and apnea along with the normal capnogram on the top.

Monitoring of Ventilation by Auscultation with a Bluetooth Pretracheal Stethoscope

Although devices that allow auscultation of breath sounds have been available for decades, their use has been hampered by the tethering effect of the tubing between the earpiece and the stethoscope bell. Advancements in technology have now made it possible to overcome this encumbrance. State-of-the-art pretracheal stethoscopes now incorporate both Piezo microphones (Fig. 44), which pick up the qualities of breath sounds with high fidelity and little background noise, as well as Bluetooth technology (Fig. 45) to eliminate the need for any connection between the operator and the sensing device (Sedation Resource, Texas, USA). With the ability to monitor the quality of breath sounds with such high fidelity, the anesthesia provider has an opportunity to assess potential airway threats as they develop, often before the adverse respiratory event becomes apparent on the capnographic tracing. For example, a faint gurgling sound often heralds the buildup of secretions that may precipitate a laryngospasm, and mild wheezing and other adventitial breath sounds can be detected before a full bronchospasm develops. Both the depth and rate of breathing as well as cessation of breathing are immediately

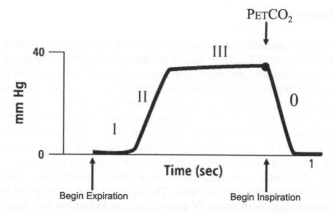

Fig. 42 The normal capnogram with its 4 phases. 0: Inspiration I: Beginning of expiration with baseline reading of 0 since atmospheric air and dead space air contain little CO_2. II: Release of CO_2 rich alveolar air leads to the rapid rise in CO_2 concentration. III: Later portion of exhalation reflecting largely alveolar gas. The dot at the end of expiration marks the $EtCO_2$. (Krauss B, Hess DR. Capnography for procedural sedation and analgesia in the emergency department. Ann Emerg Med 2007;50(2):172–81; with permission.)

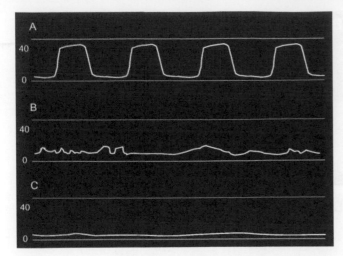

Fig. 43 Common capnographic patterns encountered in an open system typical of an outpatient OMS practice. (*Top to bottom*) Normal ventilation, alveolar hypoventilation, apnea. (*From* Lightdale JR, Goldmann DA, Feldman HA, et al. Microstream capnography improves patient monitoring during moderate sedation: a randomized, controlled trial. Pediatrics 2006;117(6):1172; with permission.)

apparent before these events are picked up by the capnograph, and long before a change in oxygen saturation becomes apparent. In addition, there is sufficient radiation of the sound of carotid pulsation that the rate and quality of heart sounds can be appreciated as well.

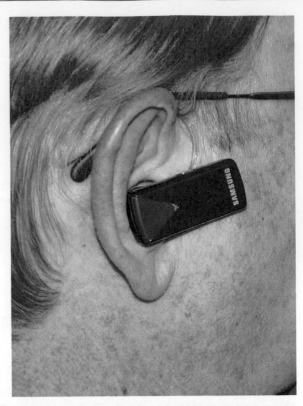

Fig. 45 The Bluetooth earpiece. The earpiece is lightweight and can be placed around glasses as well as protective goggles. (*Courtesy of* Richard C. Robert, DDS, MS, South San Francisco, CA.)

The traditional earpiece and stethoscope connection tubing can be uncomfortable to use and restricts surgeon movements. The introduction of Bluetooth wireless technology has now made the pretracheal stethoscopes user-friendly. Bluetooth headsets can be paired with an amplifier to which external speakers can also be attached if the anesthesia team wish to have the breath sounds broadcast throughout the operatory (see Fig. 9).

Summary

The first decade of the twenty-first century witnessed several advancements in office-based anesthesia for OMS. These advancements include changes in agents delivered, the manner in which they are administered, perioperative management, and monitoring. This article has dealt with some of the more significant of these changes, primary among which has been the transition of the primary anesthetic from methohexital to propofol. The rapid onset and offset of propofol accompanied by a minimal tendency to precipitate laryngospasms, as well as its antiemetic and postoperative euphoric properties, have been responsible for this shift. The agent is now often given in combination with other IV agents such as ketamine and remifentanil to provide a more balanced approach. Although the incremental bolus technique is still the most commonly used, infusion pumps have gained popularity in some offices for deep sedation and general anesthesia.

Angiocatheters have largely replaced rigid metal needles for IV access, and most patients receive a continuous IV infusion of fluid during their procedures. Much attention has been addressed at special patient populations, including those with obesity, OSA, and GERD. Emphasis has been placed on airway

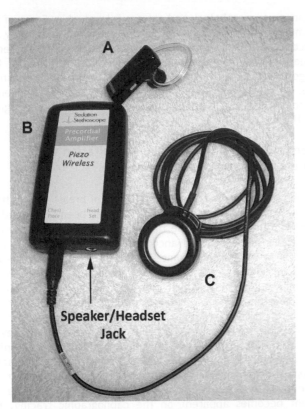

Fig. 44 The Bluetooth pretracheal stethoscope. (*A*) The Bluetooth earpiece. (*B*) Amplifier with jacks for the Piezo microphone as well as an external speaker or headset. (*C*) The pretracheal Piezo microphone. (*Courtesy of* Richard C. Robert, DDS, MS, South San Francisco, CA.)

management using nasopharyngeal airways, LMAs and tongue traction sutures.

Following the lead of the American Society of Anesthesiologists, the AAOMS has now mandated use of capnography for patients undergoing office-based anesthesia, which will become effective in January, 2014. Monitoring of ventilation has also been enhanced by technologic advances, including Piezo microphones and wireless Bluetooth adaptations for pretracheal auscultation. Some of the advancements addressed in this article have already resulted in a decrease of professional liability claims. This finding suggests that these advancements hold promise for greater safety and comfort for patients undergoing office-based anesthesia in OMS.

References

1. Perrott DH, Yuen JP, Andresen RV, et al. Office-based ambulatory anesthesia: outcomes of clinical practice of oral and maxillofacial surgeons. J Oral Maxillofac Surg 2003;61(9):983–95.
2. Vanlersberghe C, Camu F. Propofol. Handb Exp Pharmacol 2008;(182):227–52.
3. Sinner B, Graf BM. Ketamine. Handb Exp Pharmacol 2008;(182):313–33.
4. Gan TJ. Pharmacokinetic and pharmacodynamic characteristics of medications used for moderate sedation. Clin Pharmacokinet 2006;45(9):855–69.
5. Beers R, Camporesi E. Remifentanil update: clinical science and utility. CNS Drugs 2004;18(15):1085–104.
6. Handa F, Tanaka M, Nishikawa T, et al. Effects of oral clonidine premedication on side effects of intravenous ketamine anesthesia: a randomized, double-blind, placebo-controlled study. J Clin Anesth 2000;12(1):19–24.
7. Bennett J, Shafer DM, Efaw D, et al. Incremental bolus versus a continuous infusion of propofol for deep sedation/general anesthesia during dentoalveolar surgery. J Oral Maxillofac Surg 1998;56(9):1049–53.
8. Cillo Jr JE. Analysis of propofol and low-dose ketamine admixtures for adult outpatient dentoalveolar surgery: a prospective, randomized, positive-controlled clinical trial. J Oral Maxillofac Surg 2012;70(3):537–46.
9. Bennett J, Mcdonald T, Lieblich S, et al. Perioperative rehydration in ambulatory anesthesia for dentoalveolar surgery. Oral Surg Oral Med Oral Pathol Oral Radiol Endod 1999;88(3):279–84.
10. Cruthirds D, Sims PJ, Louis PJ. Review and recommendations for the prevention, management, and treatment of postoperative and postdischarge nausea and vomiting. Oral Surg Oral Med Oral Pathol Oral Radiol 2013;115(5):601–11.
11. Scuderi PE. Pharmacology of antiemetics. Int Anesthesiol Clin 2003;41(4):41–66.
12. Melton MS, Klein SM, Gan TJ. Management of postdischarge nausea and vomiting after ambulatory surgery. Curr Opin Anaesthesiol 2011;24(6):612–9.
13. Todd DW. Anesthetic considerations for the obese and morbidly obese oral and maxillofacial surgery patient. J Oral Maxillofac Surg 2005;63(9):1348–53.
14. Ingrande J, Lemmens HJ. Dose adjustment of anaesthetics in the morbidly obese. Br J Anaesth 2010;105(Suppl 1):i16–23.
15. Ankichetty S, Chung F. Considerations for patients with obstructive sleep apnea undergoing ambulatory surgery. Curr Opin Anaesthesiol 2011;24(6):605–11.
16. Hillman DR, Platt PR, Eastwood PR. Anesthesia, sleep, and upper airway collapsibility. Anesthesiol Clin 2010;28(3):443–55.
17. Puig I, Calzado S, Suarez D, et al. Meta-analysis: comparative efficacy of H2-receptor antagonists and proton pump inhibitors for reducing aspiration risk during anaesthesia depending on the administration route and schedule. Pharmacol Res 2012;65(4):480–90.
18. Khan ZH, Mohammadi M, Rasouli MR, et al. The diagnostic value of the upper lip bite test combined with sternomental distance, thyromental distance, and interincisor distance for prediction of easy laryngoscopy and intubation: a prospective study. Anesth Analg 2009;109(3):822–4.
19. Cullen DJ. Obstructive sleep apnea and postoperative analgesia—a potentially dangerous combination. J Clin Anesth 2001;13(2):83–5.
20. Barrett K, Boitano S, Barman S, et al. Ganong's review of medical physiology. 24th edition. New York: McGraw-Hill; 2012.
21. Choi SJ, Ahn HJ, Yang MK, et al. Comparison of desaturation and resaturation response times between transmission and reflectance pulse oximeters. Acta Anaesthesiol Scand 2010;54(2):212–7.
22. Nagler J, Krauss B. Capnography: a valuable tool for airway management. Emerg Med Clin North Am 2008;26(4):881–97, vii.
23. Jaffe MB. Infrared measurement of carbon dioxide in the human breath: "breathe-through" devices from Tyndall to the present day. Anesth Analg 2008;107(3):890–904.
24. Krakowiak P. Capnography—the new standard of monitoring in the OMS operatory. The Compass Newsletter. California Association of Oral and Maxillofacial Surgeons 2012. XIV:16;2.

An Office-Based Approach to the Diagnosis and Management of Osteonecrosis

Salvatore L. Ruggiero, DMD, MD, FACS [a,b,*]

KEYWORDS

- Osteonecrosis • Bisphosphonate-related necrosis of the jaw • Jaw necrosis • Bisphosphonates • Bone remodeling

KEY POINTS

- Osteonecrosis has a variable presentation related to the type of medication, duration of the medication, and the patient's concomitant medications and illnesses.
- Oral surgeons need to recognize the various stages, and provide care based on known outcomes.
- Prevention of necrosis is critical by avoiding invasive therapy and providing preemptive care before these drugs are started.

The widespread use of bisphosphonates and other antiresorptive agents as an inhibitor of bone resorption is directly attributable to their efficacy in improving the quality of life for patients with metastatic bone cancer and osteoporosis. As a potent suppressor of osteoclast activity, bisphosphonates slow the remodeling process and increase bone mineral density, thereby reducing the risk of fracture in women with osteopenia and osteoporosis.[1,2] All bisphosphonates currently approved for osteoporosis treatment have been shown to significantly reduce the risk of osteoporotic fractures. The efficacy of intravenous bisphosphonates in decreasing osteoclast-mediated lysis of bone in disease secondary to multiple myeloma, advanced breast cancer, and other solid tumors has been well established in clinical trials.[3–10] Therefore, intravenous bisphosphonates are frequently administered to patients with osteolytic metastases on a monthly basis, especially if there is a risk for significant morbidity. Based on clinical practice guidelines established by the American Society of Clinical Oncology, the use of bisphosphonates is considered the standard of care for treatment of (1) moderate to severe hypercalcemia associated with malignancy; and (2) metastatic osteolytic lesions associated with breast cancer and multiple myeloma in conjunction with antineoplastic chemotherapeutic agents.[11,12] The Food and Drug Administration has broadened the indications for intravenous bisphosphonates to include bone metastases from any solid tumor. In 2005 it was estimated that more than 2.8 million patients with cancer worldwide had received intravenous bisphosphonates since their introduction to the marketplace.[13]

Denosumab (Prolia, Xgeva) is a new antiresorptive agent that exists as a fully humanized antibody against RANK-L. As such, it is a profound inhibitor of osteoclast function and bone remodeling.

It is interesting that these agents do not bind to bone and that their effects on bone remodeling are reversible within 6 months of treatment cessation (in contrast to the bisphosphonates). The efficacy of these novel agents in preventing skeletal morbidity in patients with osteoporosis and cancer has been well established.[14–17] Unfortunately, because these agents are potent inhibitors of bone remodeling, they have also been associated with jaw necrosis in recent case reports.[18–20]

Screening

Although it was not the case 10 years ago, bisphosphonate-related osteonecrosis of the jaw (BRONJ) is now a well-recognized entity that is associated with several risk factors that have been identified across various disciplines in medicine and dentistry. Multiple risk factors including drug-related issues (potency and duration of exposure), local risk factors (dentoalveolar surgery), local anatomy, concomitant oral and systemic disease, demographic factors, and genetic factors have all been considered for this complication. Three risk factors have remained constant throughout most clinical studies:

1. Recent dentoalveolar trauma; this is the most prevalent and consistent risk factor.[21–24] Patients with a history of inflammatory dental disease (eg, periodontal and dental abscesses) are at a 7-fold increased risk for developing osteonecrosis of the jaw (ONJ).[25]
2. The duration of bisphosphonate therapy also appears to be strongly related to the likelihood of developing necrosis, with longer treatment regimens associated with a greater risk of developing disease.[23,25]
3. In addition, the more potent intravenous bisphosphonates that are administered on a monthly schedule, such as zoledronic acid and pamidronate, bind avidly to bone in high concentrations and are significantly more problematic in comparison with other preparations.

As a result of this increased awareness, medical specialists and general dental practitioners are becoming more involved in

Disclosures: Dr Ruggiero is a consultant for Amgen Inc.

[a] Division of Oral and Maxillofacial Surgery, Hofstra North Shore/LIJ School of Medicine, 270-05 76th Avenue, New Hyde Park, Hempstead, NY 11040, USA

[b] Department of Oral and Maxillofacial Surgery, Stony Brook School of Dental Medicine, Stony Brook, NY 11790, USA

* Corresponding author. New York Center of Oral and Maxillofacial Surgery, 2001 Marcus Avenue, Suite N10, Lake Success, NY 11042, USA.

E-mail address: drruggiero@nycoms.com

Atlas Oral Maxillofacial Surg Clin N Am 21 (2013) 167–173
1061-3315/13/$ - see front matter © 2013 Elsevier Inc. All rights reserved.
http://dx.doi.org/10.1016/j.cxom.2013.05.004

promoting preventive strategies for their patients at risk, which has created a greater frequency of referrals to oral and maxillofacial surgeons' offices for pretreatment screenings and risk assessment. These initial screenings can be categorized into 2 broad groups of patients based on the type of antiresorptive treatment that is anticipated. For those patients with osteoporosis or osteopenia who are about to begin oral bisphosphonate therapy there is no immediate concern, based on the fact that these patients assume a relatively small risk only after receiving these medications for longer than 3 years. These patients may proceed with dentoalveolar surgery; however, they should be educated about the risk they will assume if their antiresorptive treatment extends beyond 3 years. One notable exception applies to those patients receiving concomitant chronic long-term steroid therapy whereby the risk of necrosis may arise after a shorter duration of exposure.

For those patients receiving once-yearly dosing of zoledronic acid (Reclast) the risk of developing necrosis seems to be negligible through 3 years of treatment, based on initial studies.[26] However, the risk of necrosis for patients receiving zoledronic acid for longer than 3 years or for those receiving biannual subcutaneous denosumab remains unknown. In assessing these patients it is important to realize that most were receiving oral bisphosphonates before initiating zoledronic acid or denosumab treatments, which must be taken into consideration.

Efforts to assess risk by measuring fluctuations in bone turnover markers (eg, C-terminal telopeptide levels) are problematic and remain controversial.[27–31] The rationale for this approach is based on the knowledge that markers for bone remodeling will increase within months following withdrawal of oral bisphosphonate medications, thereby suggesting that osteoclast function and bone remodeling is normalizing.[32,33] However, these markers are a reflection of total bone turnover throughout the entire skeleton and are not specific to the maxilla or mandible, where it is suspected that the bone turnover rate may be more severely depressed from prolonged bisphosphonate exposure. From a more practical perspective, using bone-turnover markers to estimate the level of bone-turnover suppression is only meaningful when compared with baseline, pretreatment levels, which are rarely obtained in clinical practice.

A more promising mode of risk assessment may be present at the gene level. In one study certain genetic irregularities (ie, single-nucleotide polymorphisms) in the cytochrome P450-2C gene were identified in multiple myeloma patients with ONJ.[34] Those patients who were homozygous for the T allele had a 12.7-fold increased risk of developing ONJ.

Patients with cancer who are about to receive monthly treatments with zoledronic acid or denosumab will assume a measurable risk of developing jaw necrosis within a relatively short period. Management strategies similar to osteoradionecrosis prevention protocols should be implemented for such patients. The initiation of monthly intravenous or subcutaneous therapy should be delayed, if possible, until the dental health is optimized. Specifically, nonrestorable teeth and those with a poor prognosis should be extracted before the initiation of therapy. Antiresorptive therapy may begin once there is clinical evidence of bone healing at the surgical sites. Regardless of the clinical scenario, dental prophylaxis, caries control, and conservative restorative dentistry should be continued indefinitely for all patients receiving these medications. The importance of proper dental health maintenance should be underscored for all patients about to receive an antiresorptive agent, so that dentoalveolar surgery (ie, extractions, implants) can be avoided as

the risk develops in the future following extended antiresorptive medication exposure.

If antiresorptive potency, duration of exposure, and dentoalveolar surgery are true risk factors for this complication, modification of these clinical variables should translate into a reduction of disease. For those patients who are at risk of developing BRONJ, adherence to risk-reduction protocols have resulted in a decreased incidence of this complication at certain institutions.[35] Implementation of a detailed dental assessment and the avoidance of dentoalveolar surgery during treatment with zoledronic acid resulted in a 5-fold reduction of osteonecrosis.[36] In those instances where BRONJ has developed, instituting stage-specific treatment protocols has resulted in a good level of disease and symptom control in a large majority of cases (Fig. 1).[37] At several institutions, dose-reduction schedules for zoledronic acid in the setting of cancer treatment have been implemented in an effort to reduce the incidence of BRONJ while remaining oncologically effective.

Diagnosis

The American Association of Oral and Maxillofacial Surgeons established a working definition for BRONJ, which has remained unchanged since it was first defined in 2006. The tenets of the diagnosis include: (1) an exposure history to bisphosphonates, (2) exposed bone within the oral cavity, and (3) no history of prior radiation therapy to the jaws. The emergence of jaw necrosis in bisphosphonate-naïve patients receiving RANKL (receptor activator of nuclear factor κB ligand) inhibitors[14,18–20] may necessitate a modification of these criteria in the near future. Most recently the American Dental Association has introduced the more generic term ARAONJ (antiresorptive associated ONJ) in order to include those new cases of necrosis associated with monoclonal therapy. Despite the variations in nomenclature, the clinical finding of exposed, necrotic bone remains the consistent hallmark of the diagnosis and, therefore, the physical examination is the most effective method of establishing the diagnosis of jaw necrosis.

The differential diagnosis of BRONJ should exclude other common clinical conditions that may include, but are not limited to, alveolar osteitis, sinusitis, and gingivitis/periodontitis. In those rare situations where exposed bone is present in patients exposed to both bisphosphonates and radiation therapy to the jaw, osteoradionecrosis should be strongly considered. Although bone inflammation and infection is typically present in patients with advanced ONJ, this is secondary event. The exposed bone and surrounding soft tissue become secondarily infected, presenting a clinical scenario similar to that of osteomyelitis. The development of biofilms on the surface of the exposed bone has been well described and may account for the poor response to systemic antimicrobial therapy in certain patients.[38] The histologic analysis of these exposed bone specimens typically reveal necrotic bone with associated bacterial debris and granulation tissue (similar to osteomyelitis). The necrotic bone specimens do not demonstrate any microscopic features that are unique or diagnostic for BRONJ. Therefore, the role of bone biopsy in establishing the diagnosis of this condition is very limited, but may be helpful in certain rare clinical scenarios where other conditions such as metastatic or primary malignant disease must be ruled out. Analysis of the physical properties of the resected necrotic bone has also failed to demonstrate any unique features that would serve as a reliable biomarker for this disease process.[39,40]

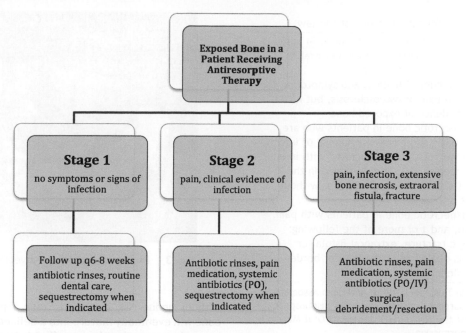

Fig. 1 Stage-specific treatment algorithm for osteonecrosis of the jaw. IV, intravenous; PO, by mouth. (*From* Ruggiero SL. Emerging concepts in the management and treatment of osteonecrosis of the jaw. Oral Maxillofac Surg Clin North Am 2013;25:11–20; with permission.)

The patient's history and clinical examination remain as the most sensitive diagnostic tools for this condition. Areas of exposed and necrotic bone may remain asymptomatic for weeks, months, or even years. These lesions are most frequently symptomatic when surrounding tissues become inflamed or there is clinical evidence of infection. Signs and symptoms that may occur before the development of clinically detectable osteonecrosis include pain, tooth mobility, mucosal swelling, erythema, and ulceration. These symptoms may occur spontaneously, or more commonly at the site of prior dentoalveolar surgery. Most case series have described this complication at regions of previous dental surgery (ie, extraction sites); however, exposed bone has also been reported in patients with no history of trauma or in edentulous regions of the jaw. Intraoral and extraoral fistulas may develop when necrotic jawbone becomes secondarily infected. Some patients may also present with complaints of altered sensation in the affected area as the neurovascular bundle becomes compressed from the inflamed surrounding bone. Chronic maxillary sinusitis secondary to osteonecrosis with or without an oral-antral fistula can be the presenting symptom in patients with maxillary bone involvement.

The radiographic features of BRONJ remain relatively nonspecific. In fact, plain radiography does not typically demonstrate any abnormality in the early stages of the disease because of the limited degree of decalcification that is present. However, findings on plain film imaging such as localized or diffuse osteosclerosis or a thickening of the lamina dura may be predictors for future sites of exposed, necrotic bone. Little or no ossification at a previous extraction site may also represent an early radiographic indication of disease. The findings on computed tomography (CT) are also nonspecific, but this modality is significantly more sensitive to changes in bone mineralization and therefore is more likely to demonstrate areas focal sclerosis, thickened lamina dura, early sequestrum formation, and presence of reactive periosteal bone. CT images have also proved to be more accurate in delineating the extent of disease, which is very helpful for surgical treatment planning.[41,42]

The utility of nuclear bone scanning in patients at risk of BRONJ has received growing attention following reports of increased tracer uptake in regions of the jaws that subsequently developed necrosis.[43,44] Although nuclear imaging has limited value in patients with existing disease, its usefulness as a predictive tool in those patients with preclinical disease (Stage 0) may have some potential benefit, and therefore requires continued evaluation.

Staging and treatment

A clinical staging system for BRONJ, implemented in 2006[45] and updated in 2009,[46] has served to categorize patients with BRONJ, direct rational treatment guidelines, and collect data to assess the prognosis and treatment outcome in patients who have used either intravenous or oral bisphosphonates (Table 1). Since the publication of these treatment guidelines, reports of nonspecific signs and symptoms such as pain, abscess formation, altered sensory function, or osteosclerosis have emerged in patients with a bisphosphonate exposure history but no clinical evidence of necrosis (Fig. 2). In an effort to determine whether these findings represent a precursor for clinical disease, the 2009 American Association of Oral and Maxillofacial Surgeons position paper has included these patients in a new category, Stage 0.[46] The degree to which patients with Stage 0 disease progress to overt ONJ remains to be determined, and represents an important area for future investigations. Recent reports in the European literature have described a variant of ONJ whereby there is bone pain with no exposed bone.[47] Of interest, more than 50% of these patients developed exposed bone at these sites within 5 months. Therefore, it seems prudent to follow these patients expectantly and reinforce the importance of dental surveillance as they continue their antiresorptive therapy.

Table 1 Staging system for osteonecrosis of the jaw

At risk category	No apparent exposed/necrotic bone in patients who have been treated with either oral or intravenous bisphosphonates
Stage 0	Nonspecific clinical findings and symptoms such as jaw pain or osteosclerosis, but no clinical evidence of exposed bone
Stage 1	Exposed/necrotic bone in patients who are asymptomatic and have no evidence of infection
Stage 2	Exposed/necrotic bone associated with infection as evidenced by pain and erythema in the region of the exposed bone with or without purulent drainage
Stage 3	Exposed/necrotic bone in patients with pain, infection, and 1 or more of the following: pathologic fracture, extraoral fistula, or osteolysis extending to the inferior border or sinus floor

From Ruggiero S, Dodson T, Assael L, et al. American Association of Oral and Maxillofacial Surgeons position paper on bisphosphonate-related osteonecrosis of the jaws: 2009 update. J Oral Maxillofac Surg 2009;67:11; with permission.

Stage 1

Patients with Stage 1 disease have exposed bone but are asymptomatic. There is no evidence of inflammatory swelling or infection of adjacent soft tissue (Fig. 3). The exposed bone is typically located at the alveolar crest but can present anywhere along the alveolar portion of the jaws. The treatment approach for patients with Stage 1 disease has remained primarily nonsurgical because these patients are not infected or symptomatic (see Fig. 3). Such patients are followed by the oral and maxillofacial surgeon every 3 to 4 months and are maintained on an antibiotic mouth rinse. Patients are also instructed to visit their general dental care provider at least every 4 to 6 months to ensure an adequate level of dental health. It is often necessary for the oral surgeon to discuss the diagnosis and management parameters with the general dentist so that appropriate dental care can be provided

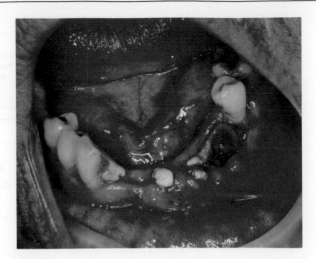

Fig. 3 Exposed, noninfected alveolar bone (Stage 1).

without undue risk. For most Stage 1 patients, the exposed bone will eventually mature into a defined sequestrum that can be easily removed within an office setting under a local anesthetic. Once the area has mucosalized, no further rinsing is required and the patient can be followed on an as-needed basis. Regardless of the stage of disease, in some patients the exposed bone can become a source of chronic irritation to the adjacent soft tissues of the tongue or floor of mouth and can cause significant pain (Fig. 4). In this instance a protective stent can be fabricated to cover the exposed bone to protect the soft tissue. In the author's experience, a more definitive approach would be to reduce and recontour the region of exposed bone with a rotary instrument and bone file under local anesthesia. The objective of this approach is not to raise a flap and remove all the adjacent bone, but rather to focus on the area that is causing the irritation. This approach minimizes the potential for additional bone exposure and necrosis, typically resulting in immediate relief of the pain and avoiding the added cost and burden of wearing an intraoral appliance.

Stage 2

Stage 2 disease is also characterized by exposed bone, but these patients present with pain and inflammatory swelling or secondary infection of adjacent or regional soft tissue (Fig. 5). Similar to patients with Stage 1 disease, these patients all

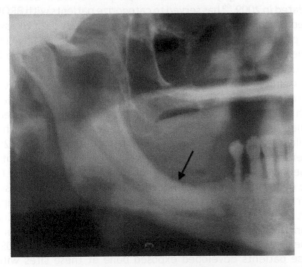

Fig. 2 Panoramic radiograph of a patient who received zoledronic acid for metastatic cancer with Stage 0. The black arrow indicates a region of osteosclerosis at the alveolar crest.

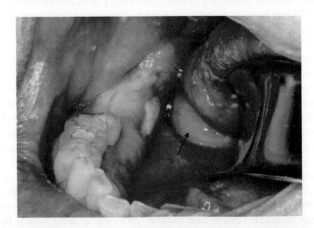

Fig. 4 Traumatic ulcer (*black arrow*) on the ventral tongue surface adjacent to exposed bone along the lingual plate.

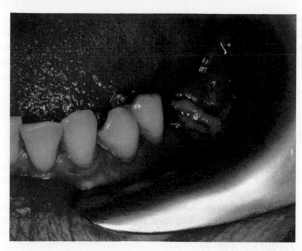

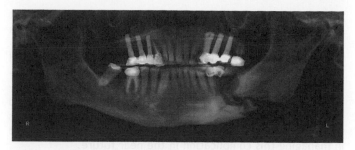

Fig. 7 Panoramic radiograph of a multiple myeloma patient with Stage 3 BRONJ and a pathologic fracture of the left mandible following 2 years of monthly zoledronic acid infusions.

Fig. 5 Exposed alveolar bone with surrounding granulation tissue and gingival inflammation (Stage 2).

require antibiotic mouth rinses and frequent surveillance. In addition, systemic oral antibiotic therapy is indicated to treat the infection and prevent a more widespread inflammatory condition. A penicillin-based regimen is typically the most effective approach because most of the pathogens are oral flora, which are penicillin sensitive. Clindamycin is an acceptable alternative for patients with penicillin allergies. In certain patients more long-term antibiotic therapy is required to suppress the chronic, recurrent nature of the infection. Doxycycline given once per day at a dose of 50 or 100 mg is usually well tolerated and can provide a more sustained, long-term level of antibiotic therapy. If there is a sequestrum at initial presentation or if it develops following antibiotic therapy or surveillance, it should be removed, leading to faster healing and reducing the need for antibiotic therapy. Depending on the size, location, and disposition of the patient, most sequestrectomy procedures can be easily accomplished in the office setting with local anesthesia. Depending on the size of the bony defect, primary closure may not be possible, in which case the wound should be left open and irrigating instructions reviewed with the patient. If a soft-tissue lining is present along the periphery of the defect it should be left intact, because it may be covering viable bone (see Fig. 5).

Stage 3

Patients with Stage 3 disease are the most challenging to manage given the extent of necrosis and the symptomatology (Fig. 6A, B). These patients have exposed bone associated with pain, inflammation or secondary infection of adjacent soft

tissue similar to Stage 2 disease, but also present with additional clinical features such as a pathologic fracture (Fig. 7), extraoral fistula (see Fig. 6B), oral-antral fistula, and radiographic evidence of osteolysis extending to the inferior border or the sinus floor. Systemic antibiotic therapy and rinses are required. Microbial cultures from areas of infected exposed bone will usually isolate normal oral microbes, and therefore are not always helpful. However, in cases where there is extensive soft-tissue involvement, microbial culture data may define comorbid oral infections that may facilitate the selection of an appropriate intravenous or oral antibiotic regimen. Patients with Stage 3 disease have an extensive degree of necrosis and infection, which usually requires early surgical treatment (segmental resection or marginal resection) for control of the infection and pain. In situations where the necrotic bone is isolated to a limited region of the maxilla, the segmental resection can be safely performed with local anesthesia in an office setting. If an oral-antral communication is anticipated, an obturator can be fabricated and delivered at the time of surgery. Larger resections of the maxilla or any segmental resection of the mandible will typically require a general anesthetic in a hospital-based operating room. For those patients who require surgical resection resulting in a continuity defect, the reconstruction can be challenging. Although there have been reports of immediate reconstruction with vascularized bone grafts, most surgeons are hesitant to proceed with such a procedure given the uncertain viability of the bone at the resection margins.[48] Alternatively, the mandibular defect can be bridged and stabilized with a reconstruction plate and soft-tissue flap that could include the condylar head if necessary (see Fig. 3).

New directions

Other approaches for the surgical and nonsurgical management for all stages of ONJ have recently emerged, and may be of

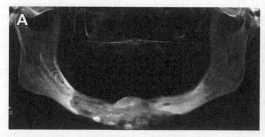

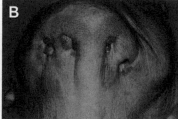

Fig. 6 (A) Panoramic radiograph demonstrating a large section of osteonecrosis extending from the body of the right mandible to the contralateral parasymphyseal region. There is necrotic bone from the crest to the inferior border (Stage 3). (B) Extraoral view of the same patient demonstrating multiple draining fistulas.

future value. Recent reports from some institutions suggest that early surgical treatment, regardless of disease stage, is associated with a predictable level of cure and disease control.[48–52] In a retrospective multicenter study that evaluated the outcomes of the surgical treatment of symptomatic patients with BRONJ, 60% of the patients who received surgery (resection or debridement) improved.[52] Those patients who were treated with resection were the most improved. This finding indicates that surgical treatment may play a larger role in managing this complication in the near future.

In a randomized prospective study of patients who received hyperbaric oxygen therapy in addition to other forms of care, the treatment group trended better in measurements of pain and quality of life score, but overall healing was reported in only 50% of patients.[53]

The use of platelet-rich plasma as an adjunct to local resection and primary closure was reported in a total of 5 cases at 2 separate institutions.[54,55] In all instances there was complete wound healing and resolution of pain; however, these studies contained a small number of cases and lacked control patients. In a small case study, systemic pentoxifylline and α-tocopherol given concurrently was found to decrease pain and the size of the exposed bone.[56] The rationale for this approach is based on other studies that demonstrated the efficacy of these drugs in the treatment of osteoradionecrosis.

Recombinant human parathyroid hormone, or teriparatide (Forteo), is the only anabolic bone agent approved for use in humans in the United States. Daily teriparatide injections stimulate enhanced bone formation through positive effects on osteoblast life span and by direct stimulation of quiescent bone-lining cells. In several case reports, the utilization of systemic low-dose parathyroid hormone was successful in resolving areas of necrosis when other modalities of treatment had failed.[57,58] In a recent prospective, placebo-controlled study of 40 patients, low-dose systemic teriparatide in conjunction with vitamin D and oral calcium was associated with greater resolution of periodontal bone defects and accelerated intraoral osseous healing.[59] These promising findings have created a new focus for future studies investigating the role of teriparatide in the prevention or treatment of this disease process. Although systemic teriparatide is currently contraindicated in patients with osteolytic bone metastases, it may have a role in the treatment of BRONJ in the noncancer setting.

Summary

ONJ that develops following exposure to antiresorptive medications remains as one of the more challenging clinical problems for oral and maxillofacial surgeons. The growing amount of data that continues to demonstrate the efficacy of antiresorptive agents (bisphosphonates, anti-RANKL antibodies) in the treatment and prevention of skeletally related events will ensure their continued use for the foreseeable future. Jaw necrosis, regardless of its cause, has remained a clinical entity that is typically diagnosed and primarily managed by oral and maxillofacial surgeons; therefore, it is important for our specialty to remain well informed about the nuances in diagnosis, treatment, and outcomes of therapy. As the level of awareness of this clinical entity broadens, the oral and maxillofacial surgeon will continue to be responsible for its primary management. The oral and maxillofacial surgeon should serve as the sentinel care coordinator for these patients, be active in the screening and risk-assessment process, and function as the primary provider of surgical and nonsurgical care. Because most patients with Stage 1 and 2 disease and certain patients with Stage 3 disease can be easily and effectively managed within an office setting, most oral and maxillofacial surgeons can manage these patients and provide easy access to much-needed care and guidance.

References

1. Chestnut C, Majumdar S, Gardner J. Assessment of bone quality, quantity and turnover with multiple methodologies at multiple skeletal sites. Adv Exp Med Biol 2001;496:95–7.
2. Guyatt G, Cranney A, Griffith L. Summary of meta-analysis of therapies for postmenopausal osteoporosis and the relationship between bone density and fractures. Endocrinol Metab Clin North Am 2002;31:659–79.
3. van Holten-Verzantvoort A, Kroon H, Bijvoet O. Palliative pamidronate treatment in patients with bone metastases from breast cancer. J Clin Oncol 1993;11:491–8.
4. Hortobagyi G, Theriualt R, Porter L, et al. Efficacy of pamidronate in reducing skeletal complications in patients with breast cancer and lytic bone metastasis. N Engl J Med 1996;335:1785–92.
5. Berensen J, Lichtenstein A, Porter L. Efficacy of pamidronate in reducing skeletal events in patients with advanced multiple myeloma. N Engl J Med 1996;334:484–93.
6. Hortobagyi G, Theriualt R, Lipton A. Long-term prevention of skeletal complications of metastatic breast cancer with pamidronate. J Clin Oncol 1998;16:2038–43.
7. Berensen J, Lichtenstein A, Porter L. Long term pamidronate treatment of advanced multiple myeloma patients reduces skeletal events. J Clin Oncol 1998;16:593–7.
8. Theriualt R, Lipton A, Hortobagyi O. Pamidronate reduces skeletal morbidity in women with advanced breast cancer and lytic lesions: a randomized placebo-controlled trial. J Clin Oncol 1999; 17:846.
9. Conte P, Coleman R. Bisphosphonates in the treatment of skeletal metastases. Semin Oncol 2004;31:59–63.
10. Michaelson M, Smith M. Bisphosphonates for the treatment and prevention of bone metastases. J Clin Oncol 2005;23:8219–24.
11. Hillner B, Ingle J, Berenson J. American Society of Clinical Oncology guideline on the role of bisphosphonates in breast cancer. J Clin Oncol 2000;18:1378–91.
12. Berenson J, Hillner B, Kyle R, et al. American Society of Clinical Oncology clinical practice guidelines: the role of bisphosphonates in multiple myeloma. J Clin Oncol 2002;20:3719–36.
13. United States Food and Drug Administration Oncologic Drugs Advisory Committee. Combidex briefing information. 2005. Accessed at http://www.fda.gov/ohms/dockets/ac/05/briefing/2005-4095b1.htm.
14. Stopeck A, Body J, Fujiwara Y. Denosumab versus zoledronic acid for the treatment of breast cancer patients with bone metastases: results of a randomized phase 3 study. Eur J Cancer Suppl 2009;7:2–8.
15. Cummings S, Martin J, McClung M, et al. Denosumab for the prevention of fractures in postmenopausal women with osteoporosis. N Engl J Med 2009;361(8):756–65.
16. McClung M, Lewiecki M, Cohen S, et al. Denosumab in postmenopausal women with low bone mineral density. N Engl J Med 2006;354:821–31.
17. Smith M, Egerdie B, Toriz N, et al. Denosumab in men receiving androgen-deprivation therapy for prostate cancer. N Engl J Med 2009;361(8):745–55.
18. Taylor K, Middlefell L, Mizen K. Osteonecrosis of the jaws induced by anti-RANK ligand therapy. Br J Oral Maxillofac Surg 2010;48:221–3.
19. Aghaloo T, Felsenfeld A, Tetradis S. Osteonecrosis of the jaw in a patient on denosumab. J Oral Maxillofac Surg 2010;68:959–63.
20. Diz P, Lopez-Cedrun J, Arenaz J, et al. Denosumab-related osteonecrosis of the jaw. J Am Dent Assoc 2012;143(9):981–4.

21. Marx R, Sawatari Y, Fortin M. Bisphosphonate-induced exposed bone (osteonecrosis/osteopetrosis) of the jaws: risk factors, recognition, prevention and treatment. J Oral Maxillofac Surg 2005;63:1567–75.

22. Durie B, Katz M, Crowley J. Osteonecrosis of the jaw and bisphosphonates [letter]. N Engl J Med 2005;353:99.

23. Badros A, Weikel D, Salama A. Osteonecrosis of the jaw in multiple myeloma patients: clinical features and risk factors. J Clin Oncol 2006;24:945–52.

24. Barasch A, Cunha-Cruz J, Curro F, et al. Risk factors for osteonecrosis of the jaws: a case-control study from the CONDOR dental PBRN. J Dent Res 2011;90(4):439–44.

25. Hoff A, Toth B, Altundag K. Osteonecrosis of the jaw in patients receiving intravenous bisphosphonate therapy. J Clin Oncol 2006; 24:8528.

26. Black D, Delmas P, Eastell R, et al. Once-yearly zoledronic acid for treatment of postmenopausal osteoporosis. N Engl J Med 2007; 356:1809–22.

27. Bagan J, Jimenez Y, Gomez D, et al. Collagen telopeptide (serum CTX) and its relationship with size and number of lesions in osteonecrosis of the jaws in cancer patients on intravenous bisphosphonates. Oral Oncol 2008;44:1088–9.

28. Kunchur R, Need A, Hughes T, et al. Clinical investigation of C-terminal cross-linking telopeptide test in prevention and management of bisphosphonate -associated osteonecrosis of the jaws. J Oral Maxillofac Surg 2009;67:1167–73.

29. Kwon Y, Kim D, Obe J, et al. Correlation between serum C-terminal cross-linking telopeptide of type 1 collagen and staging of oral bisphosphonate-related osteonecrosis of the jaws. J Oral Maxillofac Surg 2009;67:2644–8.

30. Lehrer S, Montazem A, Ramanathan L, et al. Normal serum bone markers in bisphosphonate-induced osteonecrosis of the jaws. Oral Surg Oral Med Oral Pathol Oral Radiol Endod 2008;106: 389–91.

31. Marx R, Cillo J, Ulloa J. Oral bisphosphonate-induced osteonecrosis: risk factors, prediction of risk using serum CTX testing, prevention, and treatment. J Oral Maxillofac Surg 2007;65:2397–410.

32. Rosen H, Moses A, Garber J, et al. Serum CTX: a new marker of bone resorption that shows treatment effect more often than other markers because of low coefficient of variability and large changes with bisphosphonate therapy. Calcif Tissue Int 2000;66: 100–3.

33. Rosen H, Moses A, Garber J, et al. Utility of biochemical markers of bone turnover in the follow-up of patients treated with bisphosphonates. Calcif Tissue Int 1998;63:363–8.

34. Sarasquete M. BRONJ is associated with polymorphisms of the cytochrome P450 CYP2C8 in multiple myeloma: a genome-wide single nucleotide analysis. Blood 2008;111:2709.

35. Badros A, Evangelos T, Goloubeva O, et al. Long-term follow-up of multiple myeloma patients with osteonecrosis of the jaw. Blood 2007;110(11):1030A–1A.

36. Dimopoulos M, Kastritis E, Bamia C, et al. Decreased incidence of osteonecrosis of the jaw in patients with multiple myeloma treated with zoledronic acid after application of preventive measures. Blood 2007;110(11):1056A.

37. Mehrotra B, Fantasia J, Ruggiero S. Outcomes of bisphosphonate related osteonecrosis of the jaw. Importance of staging and management guidelines. A large single institutional update. J Clin Oncol 2008;26(Suppl 20):322.

38. Kumar S, Gorur A, Schaudinn C, et al. The role of microbial biofilms in osteonecrosis of the jaw associated with bisphosphonate therapy. Curr Osteoporos Rep 2010;8:1544–2241. (Electronic).

39. Allen M, Pandya B, Ruggiero S. Lack of correlation between duration of osteonecrosis of the jaw and sequestra tissue morphology: what it tells us about the condition and what it means for future studies. J Oral Maxillofac Surg 2010;68:2730–4.

40. Allen M, Ruggiero S. Higher bone matrix density exists in only a subset of patients with bisphosphonate-related osteonecrosis of the jaw. J Oral Maxillofac Surg 2009;67:1373–7.

41. Treister N, Friedland B, Woo S. Use of cone-beam computerized tomography for evaluation of bisphosphonate-associated osteonecrosis of the jaws. Oral Surg Oral Med Oral Pathol Oral Radiol Endod 2010;109:753–64.

42. Arce K, Assael L, Weissman J, et al. Image findings in bisphosphonate-related osteonecrosis of the jaws. J Oral Maxillofac Surg 2009;67(Suppl 1):75–84.

43. Chiandussi S, Biasotto M, Cavalli F, et al. Clinical and diagnostic imaging of bisphosphonate-associated osteonecrosis of the jaws. Dentomaxillofac Radiol 2006;35:236–43.

44. O'Ryan F, Khoury S, Liao W, et al. Intravenous bisphosphonate-related osteonecrosis of the jaw: bone scintigraphy as a n early indicator. J Oral Maxillofac Surg 2009;67:1363–72.

45. Ruggiero S, Fantasia J, Carlson E. Bisphosphonate-related osteonecrosis of the jaw: background and guidelines for diagnosis, staging and management. Oral Surg Oral Med Oral Pathol Oral Radiol Endod 2006;102:433–41.

46. Ruggiero S, Dodson T, Assael L, et al. American Association of Oral and Maxillofacial Surgeons position paper on bisphosphonate-related osteonecrosis of the jaws: 2009 update. J Oral Maxillofac Surg 2009;67:2–12.

47. Fedele S, Porter S, D'Aiuto F, et al. Nonexposed variant of bisphosphonate-associated osteonecrosis of the jaw: a case series. Am J Med 2010;123:1060–4.

48. Carlson E, Basile J. The role of surgical resection in the management of bisphosphonate-related osteonecrosis of the jaws. J Oral Maxillofac Surg 2009;67(Suppl 1):85–95.

49. Mucke T, Koschinski J, Deppe H, et al. Outcome of treatment and parameters influencing recurrence in patients with bisphosphonate-related osteonecrosis of the jaws. J Cancer Res Clin Oncol 2011;137(5):907–13.

50. Stockman P, Vairaktaris E, Wehrhan F, et al. Osteotomy and primary wound closure in bisphosphonate-associated osteonecrosis of the jaw: a prospective clinical study with 12 months follow-up. Support Care Cancer 2009;18:449–60.

51. Stanton DC, Balasanian E. Outcome of surgical management of bisphosphonate-related osteonecrosis of the jaws: review of 33 surgical cases. J Oral Maxillofac Surg 2009;67(5):943–50.

52. Graziani F, Vescovi P, Campisi G, et al. Resective surgical approach shows a high performance in the management of advanced cases of bisphosphonate-related osteonecrosis of the jaws: a retrospective survey of 347 cases. J Oral Maxillofac Surg 2012;70(11):2501–7.

53. Freiberger JJ, Padilla-Burgos R, McGraw T, et al. What is the role of hyperbaric oxygen in the management of bisphosphonate-related osteonecrosis of the jaw: a randomized controlled trial of hyperbaric oxygen as an adjunct to surgery and antibiotics. J Oral Maxillofac Surg 2012;70(7):1573–83.

54. Curi M, Cossolin G, Koga D, et al. Treatment of avascular necrosis of the mandible in cancer patients with a history of bisphosphonate therapy by combining bone resection and autologous platelet-rich plasma: report of 3 cases. J Oral Maxillofac Surg 2007;65:349–55.

55. Lee C, David T, Nishime M. Use of platelet-rich plasma in the management of oral bisphosphonate-associated osteonecrosis of the jaw: a report of 2 cases. J Oral Implantol 2007;32:371–82.

56. Epstein M, Wicknick F, Epstein J, et al. Management of bisphosphonated-associated osteonecrosis: pentoxifylline and tocopherol in addition to antimicrobial therapy. An initial case series. Oral Surg Oral Med Oral Pathol Oral Radiol Endod 2010;110:593–6.

57. Harper R, Fung E. Resolution of bisphosphonate-associated osteonecrosis of the mandible: possible application for intermittent low-dose parathyroid hormone [rhPTH(1-340)]. J Oral Maxillofac Surg 2007;65:573–80.

58. Cheung A, Seeman E. Teriparatide therapy for alendronate-associated osteonecrosis of the jaw. N Engl J Med 2010;363:2473–4.

59. Bashutski JD, Eber RM, Kinney JS, et al. Teriparatide and osseous regeneration in the oral cavity. N Engl J Med 2010;363(25): 2396–405.

Extraction Socket Grafting and Buccal Wall Regeneration with Recombinant Human Bone Morphogenetic Protein-2 and Acellular Collagen Sponge

Daniel Spagnoli, DDS, MS, PhD [a],*, Christopher Choi, DDS, MD [b,c]

KEYWORDS

- Socket preservation • Socket graft • Buccal wall regeneration • Buccal wall defect • rhBMP-2/ACS
- Recombinant human bone morphogenetic protein-2 • INFUSE

KEY POINTS

- The natural evolution of the extraction socket is one of bone loss, most significantly affecting the buccal-lingual dimension.
- The healing socket regenerates through intramembranous ossification. The newly developed bone undergoes remodeling and responds to mechanical stress (modeling). The load created by a dental implant leads to long-term modeling of the bone.
- Allograft, xenograft, or alloplast grafts are static, inert materials often found unresorbed in graft sites. Residual graft particles that do not resorb can interfere with stress- and strain-induced bone modeling.
- Bone morphogenetic protein-2 (BMP-2) is a cytokine member of the transforming growth factor β superfamily that stimulates de novo bone formation. Recombinant human BMP-2 (rhBMP-2) (1.5 mg/mL) delivered via an acellular collagen sponge (ACS) is a versatile graft that can be used alone, in conjunction with mineralized cancellous particles, and with simultaneous implant placement.
- Implants placed in extraction sockets act as a construct to enhance bone regeneration. In the author's experience, implants placed in sockets with wall defects and grafting with rhBMP-2/ACS have shown excellent integration and buccal wall regeneration.
- When implant placement is not feasible, socket preservation screws can be used to support gingiva and regenerate alveolar form while maintaining biologic width.

Introduction

The long-term success and health of a dental implant relies on a viable osseous environment.[1,2] Damage to a socket can occur from infection, trauma, malpositioned teeth, or traumatic extraction, leading to an unsuitable site for implant replacement. The buccal wall is particularly important and its loss can lead to unesthetic gingival discoloration, peri-implantitis, thread exposure, and implant failure. Even in ideal situations, the normal healing process of an extraction socket is one of regressive remodeling. This process occurs from not only remodeling within the socket but also pressure from soft tissue contraction affecting the buccal wall of the alveolus. As a result, bone loss occurs more in the buccal-lingual dimension, and most significantly over the first several months.[3–6] In a systematic review, Tan and colleagues[7] reported 29% to 63% horizontal bone loss and 11% to 22% vertical bone loss 6 months after tooth extraction.

The process of socket healing has been investigated histologically and consists of a sequence that resembles intramembranous bone formation. A clot composed of erythrocytes trapped in a fibrin network is formed and stabilized immediately after extraction and over the first several days. By the seventh day, granulation tissue, or highly vascularized tissue with inflammatory infiltrate, is formed near the crestal area and the rest of the socket is filled with a provisional matrix consisting of immature mesenchymal cells, various types of leukocytes, and collagen fibers. At the end of first month, the matrix transitions to woven bone, and closure of the socket occurs with a fibrous connective layer containing keratinized epithelium. Finally, the immature bone remodels into mature lamellar bone by 2 months.[8,9] This remodeling process is characterized by a balanced interplay between osteoclastic resorption and osteoblastic formation. It continues indefinitely

Disclosures: Dr Spagnoli participated in the development of the socket preservation screw (Medtronic) and will receive royalties.

[a] Department of Oral & Maxillofacial Surgery, LSU HSC School of Dentistry, Louisiana State University, 1100 Florida Avenue, Box 220, New Orleans, LA 70119, USA

[b] Private Practice, Inland Empire Oral & Maxillofacial Surgeons, 8112 Milliken Ave Street, 102 Rancho Cucamonga, CA 91730, USA

[c] Carolinas Center for Oral & Facial Surgery, 222 East Bland Street #266, Charlotte, NC 28203, USA

* Corresponding author.

E-mail address: dspagn@lsuhsc.edu

1061-3315/13/$ - see front matter © 2013 Elsevier Inc. All rights reserved.
http://dx.doi.org/10.1016/j.cxom.2013.05.003

and is particularly rigorous in the alveolus, an area of high bony turnover.

Another important adaptive feature of bone is termed *modeling*, in which bone changes its size and shape in response to the presence and absence of external mechanical forces.[10] A dental implant under load initiates mechanotransduction pathways, specifically at the bone—implant interface. Long-term maintenance of implants involves continuous remodeling of the interface to maintain bone or replace bone that has sustained microfractures or fatigue from cyclic loading.[11] Finite elemental analysis of an osseointegrated dental implant have shown that von Mises forces are focused at the crest for angled implants (such as those in the anterior maxilla) and more evenly distributed around the implant in axially loaded implants (such as those in the posterior maxilla and mandible).[12] Thus, anterior maxillary implants are at risk of bone loss from focused forces, and thin bone if the bone is not capable of remodeling and modeling. Long-term implant survival relies on viable bone that provides a dynamic and adaptive osseous environment.

Socket grafting has become an accepted modality of preserving alveolar ridge dimensions after tooth extraction. Different techniques using various materials have been described.[13] Autogenous grafting requires a second donor site with added morbidity. Bone substitutes (allograft, xenograft, alloplast) act as a scaffold for bone formation, but histomorphometric analysis shows that the grafted site is composed of vital bone intertwined with as much as 40% of unresorbed grafting material.[14–17]

Advances in tissue engineering have enabled the reconstruction of natural form and function of missing tissues and organs. Bone morphogenetic proteins (BMPs) are members of the transforming growth factor β superfamily that are key regulators of cellular growth and differentiation. Specifically, BMP-2 has been shown to be chemotactic, and it upregulates vascular endothelial growth factor α activity and directs mesenchymal stem cells to differentiate into osteoblasts.[18]

The INFUSE bone graft (Medtronic, Memphis Tennessee) consists of genetically engineered human BMP-2, manufactured with recombinant technology. It is delivered via an absorbable collagen sponge that helps initiate clot formation and ultimately resorbs.[19] It has been shown to induce de novo bone formation (Fig. 1) and is approved by the US Food and Drug Administration for alveolar ridge augmentation for defects associated with extraction sockets.[20]

Indications
• Defects associated with extraction sockets.

Contraindications (obtained from INFUSE package insert[21])
• Hypersensitivity to recombinant human BMP-2 (rhBMP-2)/ acellular collagen sponge (ACS)
• Vicinity of a resected or extant tumor
• Presence of any active malignancy or current treatment for a malignancy
• Acute, active infection not localized to the operative site
• rhBMP-2/ACS has not been studied in an Investigational Device Exemption (IDE) trial for pediatric and pregnant patients

Preoperative planning
• Bone defects can be visualized with cone beam computed tomography (CT), but it is more often a clinical determination.

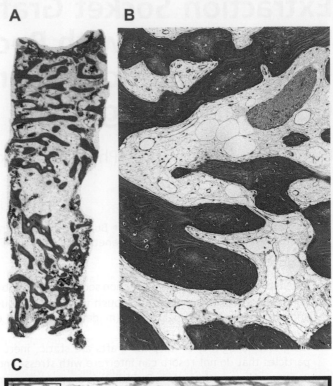
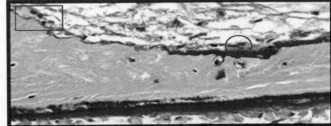
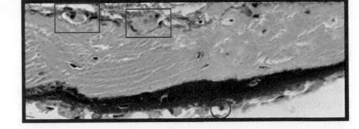
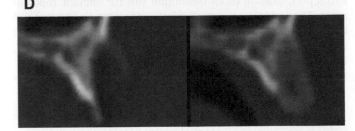

Fig. 1 Histologic sections obtained from cores of bone obtained from sockets grafted with rhBMP-2/ACS alone at 6 months. (*A*) 10× Low-power and (*B*) 25× high-power magnification (hematoxylin-eosin stain) show 100% viable bone. (*C*) Osteoclasts (*rectangle*) resorb and osteoblasts (*circle*) form bone in a process termed *remodeling*. (*D*) Computed tomography (CT) scan at baseline and 4 months after socket grafting with rhBMP-2/ACS alone show radiographic evidence of buccal wall regeneration and socket fill.

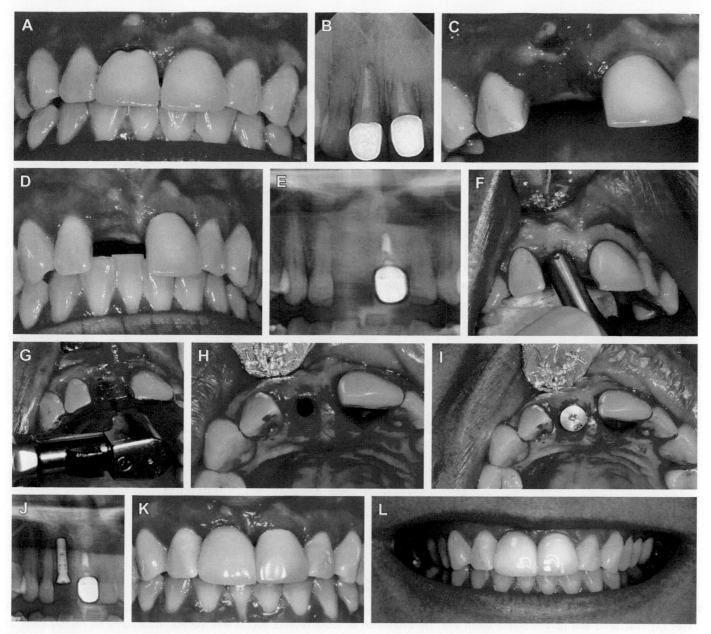

Fig. 2 Esthetic case involving extraction of tooth #8, socket grafting with rhBMP-2/ACS with mineralized cancellous particles, and implant placement at second stage. (*A*) Tooth #8 with chronic abscess after trauma with (*B*) periapical radiolucency. (*C*) Tooth #8 extracted and rhBMP-2/ACS with mineralized cancellous particles are placed into socket. (*D*) Alveolar ridge 4 weeks after extraction with homogenous bone fill (*E*) on panoramic radiograph. (*F*) Flapless surgical approach. Note excellent gingival architecture. (*G*) Use of surgical guide assists in appropriate placement. (*H*) Implant osteotomy into bleeding, viable bone. (*I*) Placement of implant with healing abutment. (*J*) Panoramic radiograph confirms implant in good position with surround bone. (*K*) Day of restoration. (*L*) Two years later with good esthetic result. Tooth #9 pending extraction.

- An XXS kit of rhBMP-2/ACS is typically sufficient to graft a socket and can be mixed with mineralized cancellous particles for added construct surface area and improved space maintenance.
- Implants can be placed immediately with rhBMP-2/ACS with good results.

Case reports
  See Figs. 2–8.

Postoperative care
- Analgesics
- Clindamycin oral rinse (900 mg diluted in 1 L of normal saline) or chlorhexidine rinse.

Potential complications
- Transient edema
- Wound dehiscence
- Loss of graft material

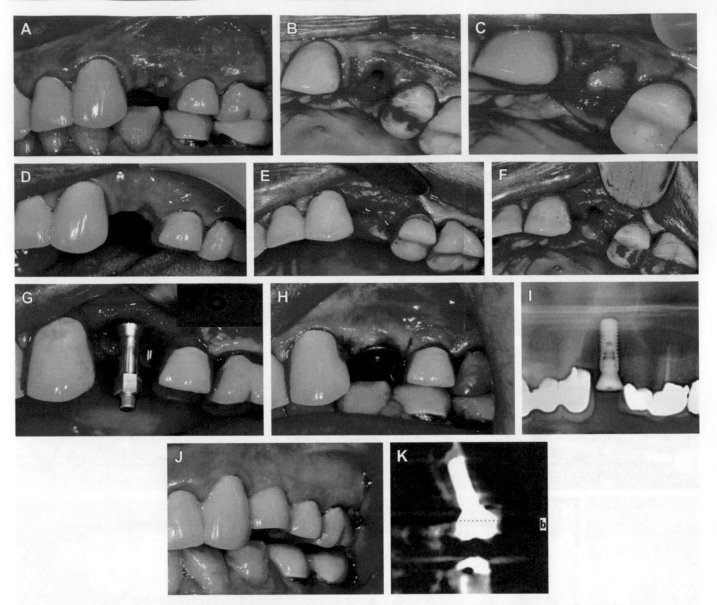

Fig. 3 Extraction of tooth #12, socket grafting and buccal wall regeneration with rhBMP-2/ACS alone, and implant placement at a second stage. (*A*) Fractured and nonrestorable tooth #12. (*B*) Extraction of tooth reveals buccal wall defect. Osteotomy on palatal bone to stimulate bleeding. (*C*) Graft with XXS kit of rhBMP-2/ACS alone. (*D*) Four months later at time of implant placement, site shows healthy soft tissue with preservation of papilla. (*E*) Surgical exposure reveals regeneration of buccal wall and (*F*) vascular bone at osteotomy site. (*G*) Implant is placed with good initial stability (Implant Stability Quotient [ISQ] value 76). (*H*) Healing abutment is placed to optimize gingival contours and papilla preservation. (*I*) Panoramic radiograph shows good position of implant. (*J*) At 8 weeks, final restoration and CT scan (*K*) shows radiographic evidence of implant osseointegration into native, viable bone.

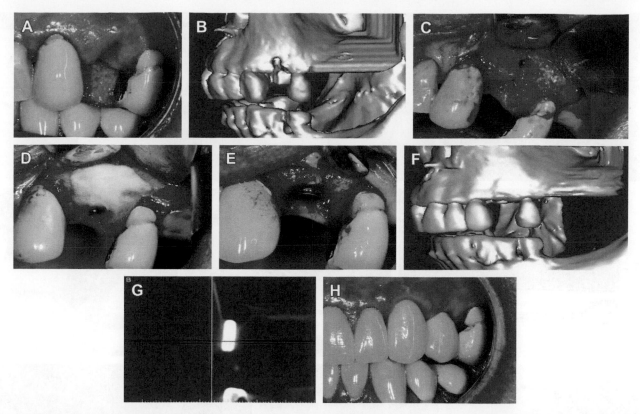

Fig. 4 Extraction of tooth #12, socket grafting and buccal wall regeneration with rhBMP-2/ACS, and immediate implant placement. This patient participated in a prospective pilot study of 6 patients that followed the same protocol detailed in Fiorellini and colleagues,[20] with the only variable being implant placement in conjunction with rhBMP-2/ACS. (A) Extraction socket with radiographic evidence of buccal wall defect on (B) 3-dimensional reconstruction of cone beam CT. (C) Surgical exposure reveals buccal wall defect. (D) Implant placed and rhBMP-2/ACS alone placed on buccal aspect. (E) 6 months later at implant uncovering, buccal wall regeneration is evident clinically and (F, G) radiographically. (H) Final restoration at 6 months as per the study protocol.[20] (*Data from* Fiorellini JP, Howell TH, Cochran D, et al. Randomized study evaluating recombinant human bone morphogenetic protein-2 for extraction socket augmentation. J Periodontol 2005;76:605.)

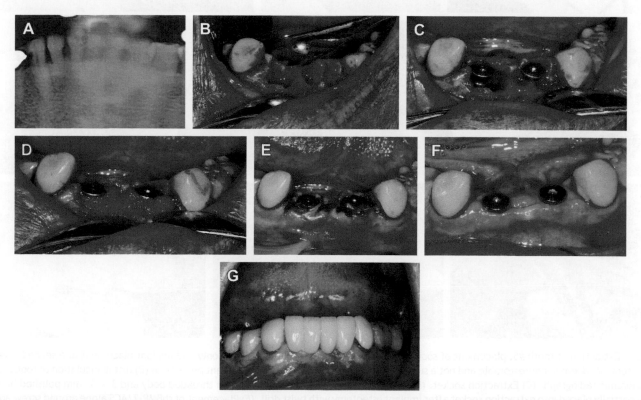

Fig. 5 Extraction of teeth #23, #24, #25, and #26; immediate implant placement; and grafting of socket defects with rhBMP-2/ACS and mineralized cancellous particles. (A) Panoramic radiograph reveals periodontal bone loss on lower anterior teeth. (B) Surgical exposure and teeth extraction reveal thin buccal bone with vertical loss. (C) Immediate implant placement in locations 23 and 26 and (D) grafting with rhBMP-2/ACS with mineralized cancellous particles. (E) Closure of soft tissue around healing abutments. (F) Twelve weeks after surgery excellent soft tissue healing is seen. (G) Three-year follow-up.

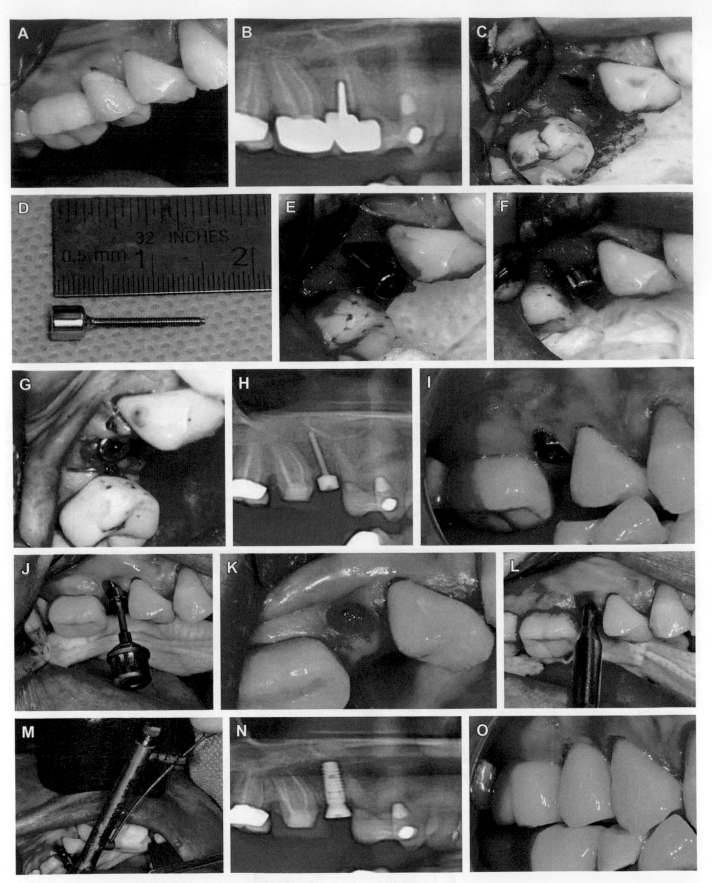

Fig. 6 Extraction of tooth #5, placement of socket preservation screw with rhBMP-2/ACS only and implant placement at a second stage. (*A*) Failing tooth #4 deemed nonrestorable and not a suitable site for immediate implant placement because of (*B*) distal angulation of tooth #5 seen on panoramic radiograph. (*C*) Extraction socket. (*D*) Socket preservation screw with 1.2-mm threaded body and 3 × 3—mm polished head. (*E*) Screw partially placed into extraction socket after implant osteotomy with twist drill. (*F*) Placement of rhBMP-2/ACS alone around screw and into socket. Head is then screwed to final depth, with base of screw placed at crestal bone height. (*G*) Closure of soft tissues around screw head, which acts like a healing abutment. (*H*) Panoramic radiograph shows good position of screw. (*I*) Five months later, gingival architecture and papilla are preserved. (*J*) Screw is removed. (*K*) Development of gingival biologic width in conjunction with socket bone regeneration. (*L*) Implant osteotome placed into screw hole. (*M*) Implant placement with torque greater than 25 Newton centimeters. (*N*) Panoramic radiograph shows implant placement in regenerated socket. (*O*) Final restoration at 2-year follow-up.

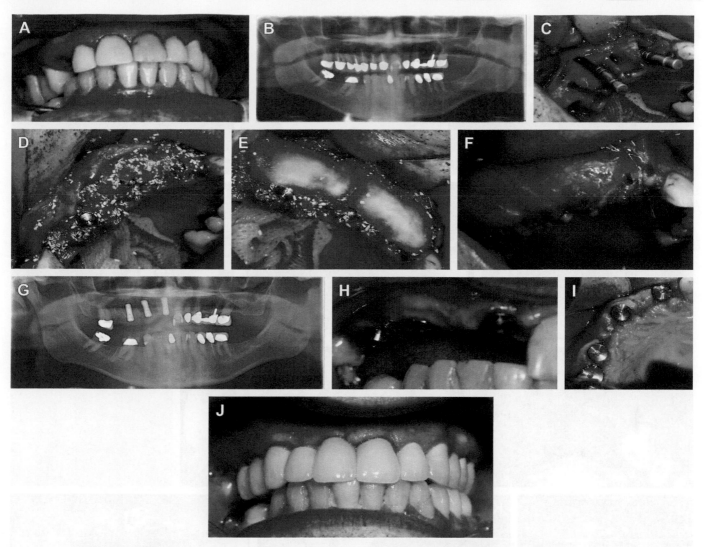

Fig. 7 Extraction of teeth #3, #4, #5, #6, #7, and #8; socket grafting and reconstruction of multiple bony defects with a trilayer graft,[22] including rhBMP-2/ACS, mineralized cancellous particles, and C-graft; and simultaneous implant placement. C-graft is derived from red sea algae and processed to develop a hydroxyapatite/tricalcium phosphate resorbable material.[23] (*A, B*) Multiple failing crowns from recurrent caries and periodontal disease. (*C*) Surgical exposure and extractions reveal multiple bony defects. Site #3 not suitable for implant placement. (*D*) Implants placed in sites 4, 6, 8 with rhBMP-2/ACS alone placed on implant surface. The space is filled with rhBMP-2/ACS and mineralized cancellous particles, and the outer wall is created by C-graft. (*E*) Strips of rhBMP-2/ACS laid on buccal aspect of graft. (*F*) Tension-free closure is obtained with chromic gut in a horizontal mattress fashion followed by oversewing with MONOCRYL in a running fashion. (*G*) Panoramic radiograph shows implant placement. (*H, I*) At 4 months, another implant is placed in site #3, and stage 2 uncovering of other implants is performed. (*J*) Final restoration at 6 months.

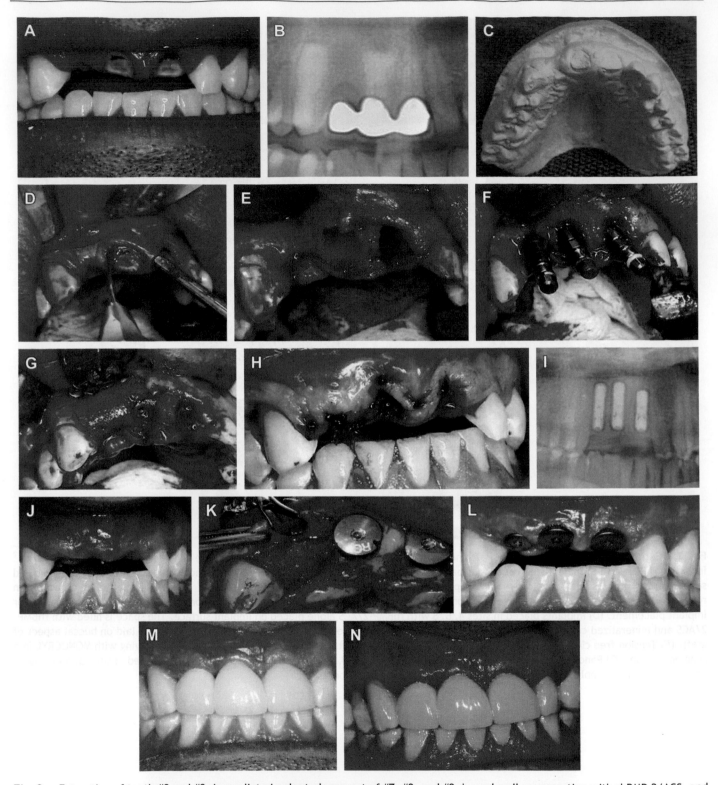

Fig. 8 Extraction of teeth #8 and #9, immediate implant placement of #7, #8, and #9, buccal wall regeneration with rhBMP-2/ACS, and high-density porous polyethylene (MEDPOR) mesh in site #7. (*A, B*) Failing 3-unit bridge with cantilever pontic in space #7. (*C*) Dental cast shows buccal concavity in area #7. (*D*) Extraction of #8 and #9 using periotome technique. (*E*) Surgical exposure reveals defect in area #7. (*F*) Implants placed in site #7 and sockets of #8 and #9. Note thread exposure on implant #7. (*G*) rhBMP-2/ACS alone is placed on buccal surface of implant and covered with MEDPOR mesh. (*H*) Closure of wound. (*I*) Two months later, panoramic radiograph shows homogenous bone fill around implants, and (*J*) soft tissue is healthy. (*K*) Removal of mesh shows osseous regeneration of buccal wall defect. (*L*) Healing after stage 2 uncovering of implants and (*M*) final restoration. (*N*) Follow-up at 1 year with good esthetic result.

Current Controversies and Future Considerations

Improved constructs based on microspinning and/or hydrogel technology will lead to improved space maintenance and growth factor delivery.

References

1. Misch CM. The use of recombinant human bone morphogenetic protein-2 for the repair of extraction socket defects: a technical modification and case series report. Int J Oral Maxillofac Implants 2010;25:1246–52.
2. Colnot C, Romero DM, Huang S, et al. Molecular analysis of healing at a bone-implant interface. J Dent Res 2007;86(9):862–7.
3. Pietrokovski J, Massler M. Alveolar ridge resorption following tooth extraction. J Prosthet Dent 1967;17:21–7.
4. Lam RV. Contour changes of the alveolar processes following extractions. J Prosthet Dent 1960;10:25–32.
5. Schropp L, Wenzel A, Kostopoulos L, et al. Bone healing and soft tissue contour changes following single-tooth extraction: a clinical and radiographic 12-month prospective study. Int J Periodontics Restorative Dent 2003;23:313–23.
6. Atwood DA, Coy WA. Clinical, cephalometric, and densitometric study of reduction of residual ridges. J Prosthet Dent 1971;26:280–95.
7. Tan WL, Wong TL, Wong MC, et al. A systematic review of post-extractional alveolar hard and soft tissue dimensional changes in humans. Clin Oral Implants Res 2012;23(Suppl 5):1–21.
8. Trombelli L, Farina R, Marzola A, et al. Modeling and remodeling of human extraction sockets. J Clin Psychopharmacol 2008;35:630–9.
9. Cardaropoli G, Araujo M, Lindhe J. Dynamics of bone tissue formation in tooth extraction sites. An experimental study in dogs. J Clin Psychopharmacol 2003;30:809–18.
10. Chen JH, Liu C, You L, et al. Boning up on Wolff's Law: mechanical regulation of the cells that make and maintain bone. J Biomech 2010;43(1):108–18.
11. Roberts WE, Smith RK, Zilberman Y, et al. Osseous adaptation to continuous loading of rigid endosseous implants. Am J Orthod 1984; 86:95–111.
12. Borchers L, Reichart P. Three-dimensional stress distribution around a dental implant at different stages of interface development. J Dent Res 1983;62(2):155–9.
13. Block MS. Treatment of the single tooth extraction site. Oral Maxillofac Surg Clin North Am 2004;16:41–63.
14. Froum SJ, Wallace SS, Elian N, et al. Comparison of mineralized cancellous bone allograft (Puros) and anorganic bovine bone matrix (Bio-Oss) for sinus augmentation: histomorphometry at 26 to 32 weeks after grafting. Int J Periodontics Restorative Dent 2006; 26(6):543–51.
15. Froum SJ, Cho SC, Rosenberg E, et al. Histological comparison of healing extraction sockets implanted with bioactive glass or demineralized freeze-dried bone allograft: a pilot study. J Periodontol 2002;73:94–102.
16. Barone A, Aldini NN, Fini M, et al. Xenograft versus extraction alone for ridge preservation after tooth removal: a clinical and histomophometric study. J Periodontol 2008;79:1370–7.
17. Cardaropoli D, Cardaropoli G. Preservation of the postextraction alveolar ridge: a clinical and histologic study. Int J Periodontices Restorative Dent 2007;28:469–77.
18. Spagnoli DB, Marx RE. Dental implants and use of rhBMP-2. Oral Maxillofac Surg Clin North Am 2011;23:347–61.
19. McKay WF, Peckham SM, Badura JM. A comprehensive clinical review of recombinant human morphogenetic protein-2 (INFUSE Bone Graft). Int Orthop 2007;31:729–34.
20. Fiorellini JP, Howell TH, Cochran D, et al. Randomized study evaluating recombinant human bone morphogenetic protein-2 for extraction socket augmentation. J Periodontol 2005;76:605.
21. Infuse package insert. Available online at http://www.medtronic. com/about-us/businesses/artificial-disc/index.htm. Accessed on July 16, 2013.
22. Buser D. Implant placement with simultaneous guided bone regeneration: selection of biomaterials and surgical principles. In: Buser D, editor. 20 years of guided bone regeneration in implant dentistry. 2nd edition. Chicago: Quintessence Publishing Co, Inc; 2009. p. 123–52.
23. Ewers R. Maxilla sinus grafting with marine algae derived bone forming material: a clinical report of long-term results. J Oral Maxillofac Surg 2005;63:1712–23.

Office-Based Management of Dental Alveolar Trauma

Richard D. Leathers, DDS [a],*, Reginald E. Gowans, DDS [b]

KEYWORDS

- Dentoalveolar trauma • Trauma treatment • Periodontal injury

KEY POINTS

- Children have a higher incidence of dentoalveolar trauma than adults.
- Injuries to the primary dentition are usually less severe and can often be managed with extractions.
- Attempts at reimplantation and stabilization of avulsed permanent teeth promptly improve outcomes.

Introduction

Literature specific to dental alveolar trauma and treatment dates back as far as the Greco-Roman period (350 BC to AD 750). Hippocrates was the first to document dental alveolar treatment regimens in his writings.[1] The concept of bridle wiring and reestablishing proper occlusion was alluded to during these early times (Fig. 1).

The causes of dental alveolar trauma are specific for age, sex, and demographics.

Age:

- Pediatric group: trauma is usually a result of falls associated with the gross weight disparity between anatomic development and skeletal weight distribution (big heads with small bodies). This type of trauma is usually seen in children aged between 2 and 4 years.
- Children in the primary dentition stage have an overall prevalence of dental alveolar trauma reaching 30%.
- Children in the mixed dentition stage have a prevalence of trauma ranging from 5% to 20%.
- Contact sports and child's play results in most of the dental alveolar trauma seen in children and adolescents.
- Child abuse is quoted in the literature as another cause of dental alveolar trauma. In the United States, more than 50% of child abuse involves trauma to the head and neck region, and internationally, 7% of injuries involve the oral cavity.
- Dental alveolar trauma in adults may involve contact sports, assaults, and motor vehicle accidents.

Sex:

- Men are twice as likely to sustain dental alveolar trauma (2:1).

Demographic:

- Most orofacial injuries resulted from intentional violence and involved primarily socially and economically disadvantaged groups in minority populations.
- Medically or psychologically challenged patients tend to be at higher risk (ie, mental, seizure, and congenital maxillofacial abnormalities).
- The most frequent general anesthesia-related litigation claim involved damage to teeth.[2,3]
- Inadequate laryngoscopy technique and the increased biting forces seen in comatose patients are another cause of dental alveolar injury (Fig. 2).[4]
- Class II division I malocclusion individuals are at risk for maxillary incisor trauma. In primary dentition, luxations (75%) are seen as opposed to crown or crown-root fractures seen in adult teeth (39%) (direct trauma).[5]
- Indirect trauma as seen in the forceful impact of the mandible with the maxilla can cause cusp injury to the posterior teeth.

When dealing with dental alveolar trauma, the standard protocol before any invasive treatment is as follows (Fig. 3):

- History and physical examination
- Maxillofacial examination
- Radiographic examination
- Standard dental alveolar trauma record
- Dental alveolar injury classification(s)
- Treatment methodology
- Pediatric versus adult treatment

History and physical examination

The ABCs (airway, breathing, circulation) are still the initial trauma norm. The patient's ABC are addressed before any dental alveolar treatment scenario.

Disclosures: The authors have nothing to disclose.
[a] Division of Oral and Maxillofacial Surgery, Harbor UCLA Medical Center, 1000 West Carson Street, Box 19, Torrance, CA 90509, USA
[b] Charles R. Drew University, 1731 E. 120th Street, Los Angeles, CA 90059, USA
* Corresponding author.
E-mail address: rleathers@dhs.lacounty.gov

Atlas Oral Maxillofacial Surg Clin N Am 21 (2013) 185-197
1061-3315/13/$ - see front matter © 2013 Elsevier Inc. All rights reserved.
http://dx.doi.org/10.1016/j.cxom.2013.05.005

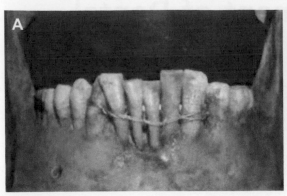
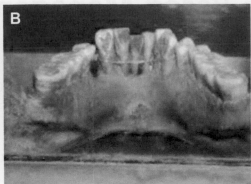

Fig. 1 Mandible found at the ancient site of Sidon in Lebanon (dated 500 BC). Gold wire was used to splint periodontally involved anterior incisors. (*A*) Frontal view. (*B*) Lingual view. (*Courtesy of* The Archaeological Museum, American University, Beirut, Lebanon; with permission.)

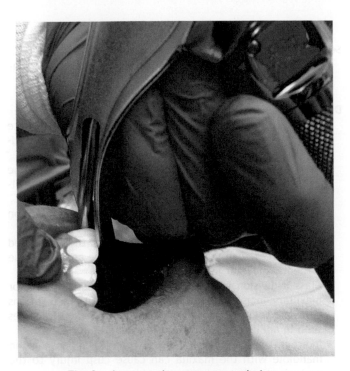

Fig. 2 Improper laryngoscopy technique.

An adequate history should include, but is not limited to, the history of the event that caused the trauma: what happened, how it happened, when it happened, and where it happened. Current occlusion and past medical history are documented. Was there a loss of consciousness (LOC)? A neurosensory deficit should be ruled out. Many dental alveolar trauma events could be substantial enough to coincidentally cause a closed head injury. Davidoff and colleagues[6,7] reported that it was not uncommon for a closed head injury to result when an LOC of less than 1 hour occurred along with facial trauma. Initial signs of confusion followed by lucid intervals could be a clue that one might require further radiographic studies (ie, computed tomography) (Fig. 4).

In initial evaluation of the dental alveolar patient, close attention to missing restorations and avulsed or fractured dentition is advised. This finding should raise the suspicion for aspiration. If these findings are noted, further radiographic

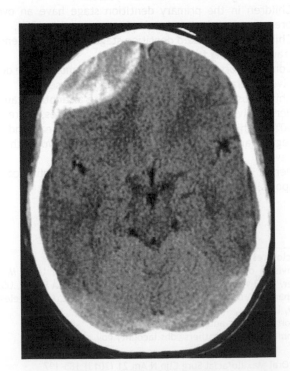

Fig. 4 Epidural hematoma.

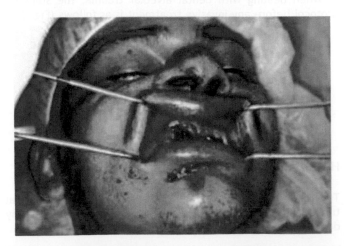

Fig. 3 Blunt facial trauma resulting in soft tissue lacerations and dental and alveolar compromise.

studies are warranted, such as neck, chest, and abdominal views. Proper follow-up and referrals should be addressed if foreign bodies are present.

Maxillofacial examination

The maxillofacial examination should be systematic and detailed. It should include but not be limited to:

- Preoperative photographs
- Extraoral cleansing
- Extraoral soft tissue
- Intraoral soft tissue
- Radiographic evaluation
- Jaws and alveolar bone
- Teeth (fractured, displacement, and mobility)
- Percussion and pulp testing
- Tetanus prophylaxis (as needed)
- Dentoalveolar trauma record

Extraoral soft tissue

Preinjury, postinjury, preoperative, and postoperative photographs can be useful both as a medicolegal tool and as a treatment goal conformational record. Successful treatment as viewed by the patient may deviate from that of the surgeon. Both are valuable assessments, which may require further treatment or referral.

Intraoral and extraoral cleansing with an antibiotic rinse (0.12% chlorhexidine) and antiseptic soap, (betadine), respectively is a mainstay before any invasive evaluation or treatment regimen. In cases of tissue continuity defects, avoid overzealous scrubbing, which may further inoculate the involved site with debris or foreign bodies.

Treatment considerations are invariably linked to the mechanism of injury. Blunt trauma or penetrating (gunshot wound, laceration) trauma defects present differently. Soft tissue laceration versus soft tissue deficit or loss may be a treatment consideration, as well as tooth fracture versus exarticulation or aspiration. Bony fracture(s) of the maxilla or mandible and temporomandibular joint (TMJ) considerations are all possibilities that may involve dental alveolar injuries.

A clinical and visual inspection of the extraoral tissues, as well as previous tetanus compliance, may indicate tetanus prophylaxis.

Intraoral soft tissue

When inspecting intraoral injuries, look for deeply penetrating soft tissue wounds, which are usually associated with a hematoma or an ecchymotic area. The lips, tongue, soft palate, buccal mucosa, and alveolar mucosa are all sites at risk for laceration or contusion injuries, depending on the mechanism of injury.

Buccal mucosal injuries should alert the surgeon of possible Stenson duct injuries and less likely cranial nerve VII involvement. Lacerations or penetration injuries of the floor of the mouth should alert 1 of Wharton duct or neurovascular injuries.

Radiographic evaluation

The most common radiographs used in dentoalveolar trauma are the periapical, occlusal, panoramic radiograph (Panorex), chest film (as needed), and abdominal film (as needed).

Periapical films are best used for tooth and root fractures; as well as luxations. These films are useful in confirmation of proper treatment protocols.

Occlusal radiographs are as effective as periapical radiographs, but provide a wider view. They can also be used more efficiently in the pediatric population. Also they have shown adequate and efficient viewing of soft tissue foreign body dislodgements.

The panoramic radiograph is probably the most useful and inclusive of the dentoalveolar films. It gives adequate views of compromise of the bony maxilla and mandible, dentition, and alveolar ridges.

Chest and abdominal radiographs, although not dentoalveolar films, become invaluable when teeth or foreign bodies are aspirated or swallowed. These structures can be accessed and followed as needed.

Jaws and alveolar bone

Step defects of the occlusion or alveolar mucosa are suspicious for maxillary or mandibular fractures. Sublingual ecchymosis is usually pathognomonic for mandibular fractures. Any form of malocclusion should further raise suspicion for fracture of the mandible. Inability to open or close adequately could be of TMJ insult. This insult is seen when hemarthrosis is present after blunt trauma to the chin, which transfers condylar forces to the eminence and causes a hematoma in the joint space (Fig. 5).

Teeth (fractured, displacement, and mobility)

Account for all luxated, fractured, or missing teeth. Consider the possibility of teeth aspirated, swallowed, or dislodged into surrounding soft tissue or sinus regions. Keep in mind the obscure nature of the indirect dental injury in which

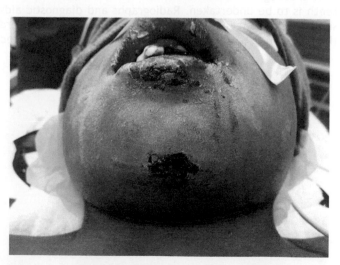

Fig. 5 Blunt trauma to the chin.

there is a blow or fall to the chin, possibly causing secondary vertical or palatal cusp fracture(s) of the maxillary bicuspids. When there is doubt, radiographic confirmation is the rule (Fig. 6).

Percussion and pulp testing

The vitality of teeth is tested via several modalities, such as thermal, mechanical, electrical, and laser. These tests may include:

- Thermal
  - Ice
  - Ethyl chloride
- Mechanical
  - Dental probe
  - Saline-laden cotton pledget
- Electrical
  - Electric pulp testers
- Laser
  - Laser Doppler flowmetry (LDF)

These tests, except LDF, can be ambiguous, because they check conduction disturbances at the sensory receptors of the pulp. The pulp comprises slowly increasing myelinated pain fibers while simultaneously lowering the electrometric pulp stimulation. These fibers regulate vascular changes and respond to pain stimuli.[8,9] The results may be erroneous because of the varying changes in myelinated verses nonmyelinated pulp fibers And also because of changes in the response caused by the slowly healing fibers during the acute phase. The acute phase may show varying results caused by revascularization in a 1-month period. False-negative results are likely during this time.[10]

When presented with both perioral and extraoral injuries, such as a lip laceration along with dental alveolar injuries, the sequence of treatment is usually the repair of the intraoral injury and then subsequent repair of the perioral lip laceration. However, if there is heavy or uncontrolled hemorrhage from the lip, this should then be addressed first.

A thorough examination of all involved and suspected teeth is to be undertaken. Radiographs and diagnostic aids should be documented in a dentoalveolar trauma record (Fig. 7). This standardized treatment record is generated

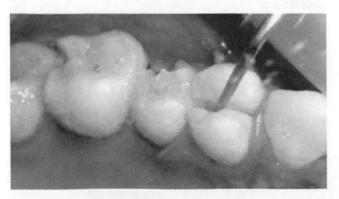

Fig. 6 Indirect dental injury.

during the evaluation process. Its goal is to aid a systematic diagnosis, treatment plan, and prognosis.

The first evaluation of teeth is visual. Is there a fracture and what is its classification? The general classifications that are well recognized are the Ellis and Davey classification (Fig. 8) and the Andreasen classification (Figs. 9–12).

The Ellis classification has 4 anatomic classes (I–IV). Class I involves fractures within enamel only, Class II involves fractures of enamel-dentin, Class III involves pulp, and class IV involves root-isolated fracture. This system involves only permanent dentition.

The Andreasen classification is a more definitive system, which was adopted by the World Health Organization, which used the International Classification of Disease codes. Ideally, this system involves both deciduous and permanent dentition. It takes into account trauma to the gingival and oral mucosa, teeth, the pulp, periodontal (PDL) tissue, and supporting structures.

The Andreasen system comprises injuries to gingival and oral mucosa, injuries to the tooth, injuries to tooth and pulp, injuries to PDL tissue, and injuries to supporting alveolar bone.

Injuries to the gingival and oral mucosa

- Abrasion
- Contusion
- Laceration

Injuries to tooth and pulp

Injuries to tooth and pulp include:

Crown infraction—a crack or craze line involving enamel only. Enhance viewing via transillumination.

Treatment: None.

Crown fracture confined to enamel and dentin—Fracture crosses the enamel-dentin border. Considered an uncomplicated fracture. No root involvement.

Treatment: Smoothing edges or repairing with composite restoration.

Crown fracture compromising pulp—Pulp exposure. Considered a complicated fracture.

Treatment: Refer for conventional root canal treatment (RCT) with future repair or full coverage restoration.

Fracture involving enamel, dentin, and cementum without pulp exposure—Considered an uncomplicated root fracture.

Treatment: Refer for build-up with full coverage crown placement.

Complicated crown-root fracture—Fracture involving enamel, dentin, and cementum, with pulp exposure. Considered complicated.

Treatment: Consider fracture position. If a coronal fracture is approximately one-third of the clinical root, consider extraction. If the fracture is closely approximating the cervical margin, then refer for RCT, crown lengthening, build up, with full coverage crown placement.

Horizontal root fracture—Treatment: Address location of horizontal fracture. If fractured at the cervical third, consider extraction versus orthodontic extrusion of the root, RCT, build up, full coverage of crown. If apical third fracture is present, monitor, no RCT, and look for interposition connective tissue at

Dentoalveolar Traum a Record

Name: _____   Date: _____

Age:

Sex:

Incident:

    Cause

    Location

    Time

Neurologic status:

    Loss of consciousness

    Consciousness

    Headache

    Nausea, vomiting

Extraoral findings:

Intraoral findings:

Radiographic findings:

    Posteroanterior

    Occlusal

    Panoramic

    Other

Tooth vitality findings (pulp testing):

Tooth mobility (+1, +2, +3):

Ellis classification (I, II, III, IV):

Luxation: Yes _____   No _____   Type _____

Avulsion: Yes _____   No _____   Storage medium _____   Time _____

Supporting structure trauma:

Diagnosis:

Treatment plan:

Prognosis: Good _____   Fair _____   Guarded _____

Examined by:

Fig. 7 Dentoalveolar trauma record.

the fracture site. This fracture usually does not require stabilization.

Injuries to PDL tissue

Injuries to PDL tissue are usually the result of some form of trauma that causes tooth movement or dislocation, with a resultant decrease or loss of the PDL space. The late complication that may result from such injuries is the development of a secondary resorptive process. This cause is essentially the same as that which is seen in the avulsion injuries. The resorption complication is classified as either root surface resorption or root canal resorption.

Root surface resorption (external root resorption)

- Surface resorption
- Replacement resorption
- Inflammatory resorption

Surface resorption is seen as exposed superficial resorption lacunae. Surface resorption is caused by injury to the PDL or

cementum. This process is essentially self-limiting and heals without incident.

Replacement resorption or ankylosis presents as root substance being replaced by bone with the loss or decrease of the PDL space.

The inflammatory resorption process presents as cementum and dentin resorption secondary to infected and necrotic pulp tissue within the root canal.

Root canal resorption (internal root resorption)

Internal replacement resorption
Internal replacement resorption presents as metaplastic replacement of pulp tissue into cancellous bone, resulting in a widened pulp chamber. This resorption is predominantly seen in root fracture injuries.

Inflammatory resorption
Inflammatory resorption is seen at the cervical region of the pulp and is caused by the ingression of bacteria via dentinal tubules within a necrotic pulp (necrotic pulp zone). This process is treated with conventional RCT.

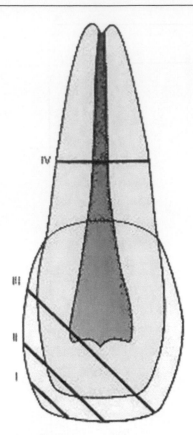

Fig. 8 Ellis classification: I = fracture within enamel; II = fractures involving the roots.

PDL injuries

PDL injuries are classified as concussions and displacements.

Concussions

Concussions consist of minimal injury to the traumatized teeth or tooth. The concussion is diagnosed by an acute hyperemic-like response to percussion in a horizontal and vertical direction.

Treatment is usually close monitoring and adjusting the traumatized tooth or opposing tooth out of occlusion.

Displacements

Displacements include luxation injuries of deciduous and permanent teeth. The teeth at highest risk are the maxillary incisors in patients with normal occlusion and the mandibular incisors for those in a class III dentofacial deformity. In the primary dentition, luxations are more prevalent, and in the permanent dentition, the injury is more likely to present as a tooth fracture. Data by Andreasen and colleagues[10] stated that 15% to 61% of luxation injuries occurred in permanent dentition and 62% to 73% occurred in primary dentition as a result of the increased elasticity in the primary dentition bony supporting structures. Luxation injuries include subluxation, intrusive luxation, extrusive luxation, lateral luxation, and exarticulations.

Subluxation

Subluxation involves an injury to the dental supporting structures that results in some degree of tooth loosening. There is no radiographic or clinical evidence of involved tooth movement; however, there is compromise to the PDL tissues, as shown by bleeding at the gingival margin.

Treatment involves occlusal adjustments, as performed with concussion injuries, and periodic involved tooth vitality testing for ~6 to 8 weeks. Consider endodontic therapy if pulpal necrosis ensues. These injuries result in external resorption approximately 4% of the time.[11]

Intrusive luxation

Intrusive luxation is associated with displacement of the tooth into the socket. It usually involves the maxillary teeth because of the less dense trabecular bone. Intrusive injuries are most severe in the pediatric population as a result of the impingement or trauma of the deciduous tooth to the tooth bud of the permanent successor in its buccal-occlusal position. This situation can often lead to hypoplasia of the facial or buccal surface (Figs. 13 and 14).[12,13] Pulpal necrosis approximates ~96%, with inflammatory resorption incidence reaching 52%.

Treatment is contingent on root development. For cases involving incomplete root development, allow for reeruption. If unsuccessful in 3 months, assist with the use of an orthodontic extruding appliance. Consider endodontic therapy if pulpal necrosis occurs. If there is complete root development, then reposition the tooth and stabilize with a nonrigid splint. Proceed with endodontic therapy in approximately 2 weeks.

Extrusive luxation

Extrusive luxation is the partial displacement of the tooth out of the socket in a coronal or incisal direction with lingual or palatal deviation of the crown. Gross mobility and bleeding at the gingival margin are noted. Radiographically, a widened PDL space is seen. Pulp necrosis occurs ~64% of the time (Figs. 15 and 16).

Treatment involves replacing the tooth in the socket. Level, align, and check occlusion. Stabilize with a nonrigid splint for approximately 2 weeks. Consider endodontic therapy in cases of pulp necrosis.

Lateral luxation

Lateral luxation usually involves traumatic forces that displace the tooth or teeth in the lingual direction. Radiographic occlusal views appear similar to that of an extruded tooth, with widening of the PDL space in the apical direction. Lingual and buccal plate expansion tendency may cause mobility of the tooth. Linear or comminuted tooth fractures are often seen, along with soft tissue compromise. Bony step defects and gingival lacerations are often seen.

Treatment involves placing the tooth or teeth back into the preinjury position and occlusion. Digitally compress lingual and buccal expansion sites to expedite PDL repair. Longer nonrigid splinting may be needed for approximately 2 to 8 weeks, depending on bony healing requirements. Any gingival or perioral lacerations should be repaired last, unless bleeding is uncontrolled or treatment is delayed because of other concomitant higher level injuries. Also, check and recheck involved tooth vitality. Consider endodontic intervention if pulpal necrosis presents. A complication that may be encountered is the loss of marginal bone support. This complication is seen clinically as an ingrowth of granulation tissue at the gingival crevice, which results in possible loss of attachment. In this case, continue splint maintenance and upgrade oral hygiene. This strategy may aid in maintaining or preventing

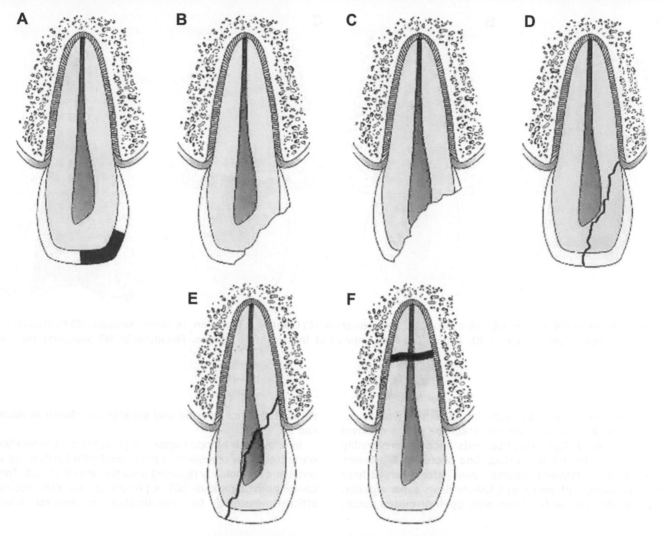

Fig. 9 Injuries to dental tissue and pulp. (*A*) Crown infraction. (*B*) Crown fracture confined to enamel and dentin (uncomplicated crown fracture). (*C*) Crown fractures directly involving pulp (complicated). (*D*) Uncomplicated root fracture. (*E*) complicated crown-root fracture. (*F*) root fracture. (*Adapted from* Andreasen JO, editor. Traumatic injuries of the teeth. 1st edition. Philadelphia: WB Saunders; 1972; with permission.)

further bone loss. The frequency of bone loss approaches 5% in lateral luxations versus 31% in intruded luxations.[14]

Exarticulations (avulsions)

The avulsion injuries are considered worst in the dentoalveolar class. These injuries involve the complete dislodgement of the tooth or teeth from the socket for a period. These injuries may require specific and tested treatment protocols to effectively limit dental compromise or loss. Areas of concern may involve potential aspiration and supporting structure loss or compromise, soft tissue trauma, or loss of the tooth or teeth. Avulsion injuries occur in both primary (7%–13%) and permanent (0.5%–16%) dentition. Children from ages 7 to 9 years are at higher risk for such injuries. The maxillary central incisors are most often at risk because of the relative instability of the PDL during their eruption phase.[10]

Treatment is based on the concept of early reestablishment of PDL cellular physiology. Decreased extraoral time and the viability of the PDL fibers that are attached to the avulsed tooth root are the goal to attain before reimplantation. Over time, many solutions have been proposed to maintain and transport avulsed teeth. The solutions that are most physiologic are Hank

solution and Viaspan (Figs. 17 and 18). The pH and osmolality of these solutions closely mimic physiologic conditions. They can store avulsed teeth and replenish cellular metabolites for 24 hours and 1 week, respectively (Table 1).

The availability and cost-effectiveness of Hank solution Save-A-Tooth make it the transport medium of choice in the storage of avulsed teeth. It is readily available in many school and athletic first-aid kits. For the lay person, cow's milk is the medium of choice in the absence of Hank solution or Viaspan; however, the pH and osmolality fall short of physiologic conditions. Milk is best served to prevent further cellular demise and is specific for teeth that have been extraoral for less than 20 minutes. It becomes ineffective after 6 hours.

The treatment course is based on several factors. Root maturation (open vs closed apex), extraoral time/medium, general health of the avulsed tooth before injury, and the supporting bone replant site.

Teeth that avulsed and present with gross decay, exposed pulp, moderate to severe PDL disease, apical abscess, supporting bone loss, or infection at the replanting site are all at higher risk for treatment failure. An alternative approach should be considered in these cases.

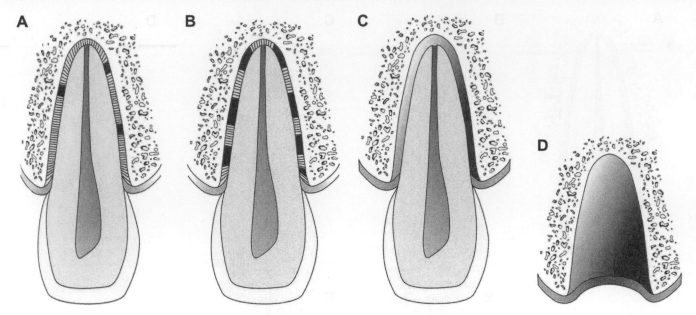

Fig. 10 Injuries to PDL tissues. (*A*) PDL concussion. (*B*) Subluxation. (*C*) Luxation, dislocation, or partial avulsion. (*D*) Exarticulation or avulsion. (*Adapted from* Andreasen JO, editor. Traumatic injuries of the teeth. 1st edition. Philadelphia: WB Saunders; 1972; with permission.)

The basic treatment to optimize success involves replantation within a 2-hour period; stabilize with a nonrigid splint for 7 to 10 days. The PDL cells become irreversibly necrotic after the 2-hour period. One should still attempt the avulsion treatment course even after this 2-hour period, knowing that treatment failure flows exponentially. The treatment course for cases with open or closed apices

within the 2-hour period and greater are shown in Boxes 1 and 2.

In cases with an open apex, an endodontic apexification is warranted. This procedure is performed with CaOH filling material and periodically replaced until the apex is closed. Then a conventional definitive RCT is performed. An alternate more efficient material for apexification is mineral trioxide

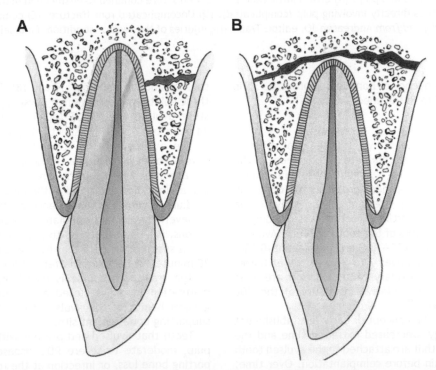

Fig. 11 Injuries to supporting alveolar bone. (*A*) Fracture of single wall of the alveolus. (*B*) Fracture of the alveolar process. (*Adapted from* Andreasen JO, editor. Traumatic injuries of the teeth. 1st edition. Philadelphia: WB Saunders; 1972; with permission.)

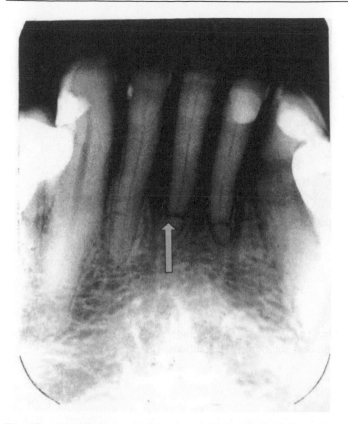

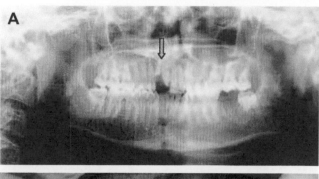

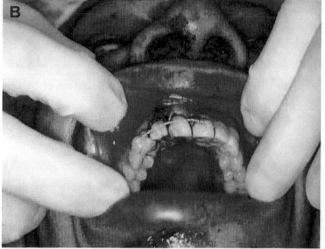

Fig. 12 Mandibular central incisors with fracture of the apical one third. No stabilization was used. Vital pulp testing was noted after 8 weeks. Note the interposition of connective tissue at the fracture site (*arrow*). (*Courtesy of* Drs Thomas G. Dwyer and James R. Dow, Roseville, CA.)

Fig. 13 (*A*) Panorex view extent of intrusion. (*B*) Teeth extruded, aligned and stabilized with nonrigid splint. Soft tissue gingival wound repaired.

aggregate. It allows for excellent tissue biocompatibility and immediate apical seal.[15]

Splinting requirements and technique

The goal of splinting in dentoalveolar injuries is to stabilize mobile teeth or bony segments into preinjury occlusion and alignment. This procedure allows for early pulpal revascularization and PDL healing course to take place. Although there are several possible techniques, the acid-etch/resin splint or variants of this splint are the treatment of choice. This technique fulfills the requirements needed in most alveolar and dental fracture injuries. Many of the other techniques may violate 1 or more of the basic treatment principles. A commonly misused technique is the arch bar splint. It is known to produce eruptive or extrusive forces on the relatively mobile tooth or segment because of its errant placement beneath the height of contour or the tooth. The splint requirements and the acid-etch technique are shown in Boxes 3 and 4.

Fractures of the alveolar process

These fractures are at a higher risk because of their exposed anatomy. Most occur in the incisor and premolar regions. The treatment course involves an early reduction and stabilization

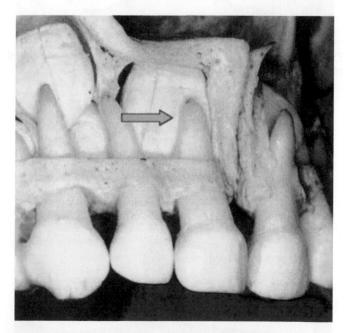

Fig. 14 Anatomic position of the primary dentition to the developing permanent tooth bud. Note the buccal-occlusal and buccal-incisal position of the primary roots (*arrow*).

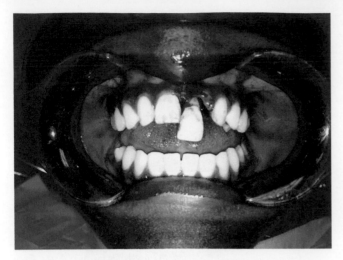

Fig. 15 Extrusive luxation with palatal deviation of crown.

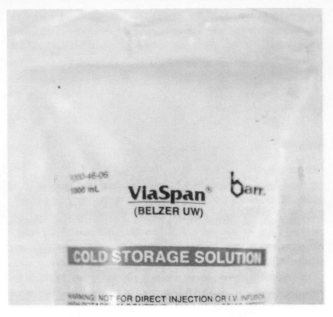

Fig. 18 Viaspan, cold storage solution available as an organ transport solution. (BTL Solutions, LLC, Columbia, SC).

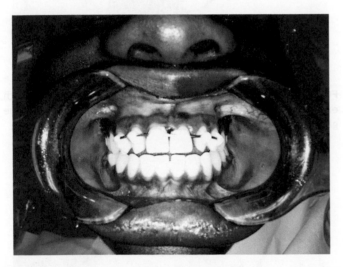

Fig. 16 Tooth level, align, checked occlusion, and splint placement.

of the involved segments. A closed or open technique may be indicated. The closed technique may involve digital manipulation and pressure along with rigid splint stabilization. This splint should remain in place for approximately 4 weeks (Fig. 19).

An open technique is indicated in cases of gross displacement and inability to freely reduce fracture segments such as that seen with root or bony interferences. Treatment involves adequate exposure of fractured segments with an incision beneath the fracture lines. Fractures are then freed up and reduced, proper occlusion and alignment attained then stabilized with transosseous wire or a small 2.0-mm monocortical miniplate. If needed, a secondary acid-etch/resin splint should be used to stabilize slightly mobile teeth in the fractured segment. The wound is then copiously irrigated with 0.9% NaCl and closed meticulously. Bony segments or hardware should not be exposed to bacterial ingression. In cases of more complex avulsive injuries, bony exposure may be evident. This situation should be approached with the aid of judicious soft tissue coverage with mucosal advancement flaps (Fig. 20).

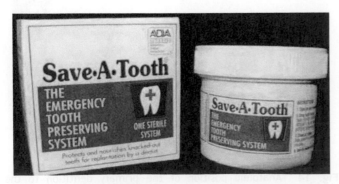

Fig. 17 Hank balanced salt solution, commercially available as Save-A-Tooth (Phoenix Lazarus).

Table 1 Solutions to replenish PDL ligament cell metabolites

Solution	Characteristics
Hank balanced salt solution	pH = 7.2 Osmolality = 320 mOsm
Viaspan	pH = 7.4 Osmolality = 320 mOsm
Cow's milk	pH = 6.5–6.7 Osmolality = 225 mOsm

Box 1. Treatment summary for avulsed teeth less than 2 hours

Open Apex
1. Replant immediately if possible
2. Transport in Hank solution or milk
3. Present to nearest qualified facility (decrease time, call first)
4. Check ABCs; evaluate for associated injuries (history and physical examination)
5. Store in Hank solution for ~30 minutes
6. Transfer to a 1-mg/20-mL doxycycline bath for 5 minutes
7. Perform radiography (posteroanterior, occlusal, panoramic, chest)
8. Initiate local anesthesia
9. Irrigate socket with 0.9% NaCl solution
10. Consider tetanus prophylaxis as needed
11. Initiate antibiotic coverage
12. Replant tooth or teeth
13. Splint 7 to 10 days (nonrigid)
14. Perform apexification CaOH in cases of pathosis

Closed Apex
1. Store in Hank solution for ~30 minutes
2. Replant tooth or teeth
3. Splint for 7 to 10 days
4. Perform endodontic cleansing and shaping of canal at time of splint removal
5. Fill canal with CaOH (6–12 months)
6. Perform final gutta-percha obturation (6–12 months)

Box 2. Treatment summary for teeth avulsed more than 2 hours: open or closed apex

1. Replant immediately, if possible
2. Transport in Hank solution or milk
3. Present to nearest qualified facility (decrease time, call first)
4. Check ABCs; evaluate for associated injuries (history and physical examination)
5. Bathe tooth in sodium hypochlorite for ~30 minutes versus manual debridement of the PDL
6. Perform extraoral RCT
7. Bathe tooth in citric acid (~3 minutes)
8. Bathe tooth in 1% stannous fluoride (~5 minutes)
9. Transfer to a 1-mg/20-mL doxycycline bath for ~5 minutes
10. Perform radiography (posteroanterior, occlusal, panoramic, chest)
11. Initiate local anesthetic
12. Perform tetanus prophylaxis as needed
13. Initiate antibiotic coverage
14. Replant tooth
15. Splint for 7 to 10 days (nonrigid)

Box 3. Splint requirements

The splint should:
1. Be able to be applied directly in the mouth without delay due to laboratory fabrication
2. Stabilize the injured tooth in the normal preinjured position
3. Provide adequate fixation throughout the period of immobilization
4. Neither damage the gingival nor predispose to caries and should allow for a basic oral hygiene regimen
5. Not interfere with occlusion or articulation
6. Not interfere with any required endodontic therapy
7. Preferably fulfill esthetic demands
8. Allow a certain mobility (nonrigid) to aid PDL ligament healing in cases of fixation after luxation injuries and replacement of avulsed teeth; however, after root fracture, the splint should be rigid to permit optimal formation of a dentin callus to unite the root fragments
9. Be easily removed without reinjury to the tooth

Adapted from Andreasen JO, Andreasen FM. Textbook and color atlas of traumatic injuries to the teeth. 3rd edition. Copenhagen: Munksgaard; 1994. p. 347–8; with permission.

Box 4. Sequence of acid-etch splinting technique[a]

1. Perform alveolar bony reduction and/or replantation
2. Perform localized cleansing and debridement
3. Isolate and dry area
4. Custom fabricate wire (~26 Ga), double-stranded monofilament nylon line, or paper clip; extend wire to at least 1 or 2 teeth on either side of the involved tooth or teeth
5. Etch the incisal half of the labial surface of the involved and adjacent teeth with gelled phosphoric acid for 30 to 60 seconds
6. Remove etchant with water stream for ~20 seconds
7. Air-dry etched surface; surface should appear chalky white
8. Passively place prefabricated wire to involved teeth
9. Stabilize splint with fast-setting autocure or light-cure composite resin
10. After resin is set, smooth rough edges with a fine acrylic or diamond finishing bur (check occlusion)
11. Perform soft tissue and gingival repair as needed
12. Remove splint in 7 to 10 days

[a] It may be prudent to use a composite shade that differs from the natural color of the teeth because this facilitate ease of removal and prevents trauma to the enamel.

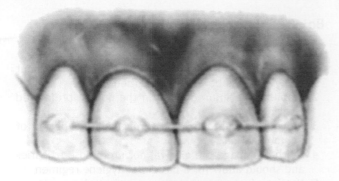

Fig. 19 Nonrigid splint.

Trauma to the gingiva and alveolar mucosa

Injuries to the gingival and alveolar mucosa mainly consist of abrasion, contusion, and laceration. These injuries can be obvious or insipient. They must be diagnosed early so as to not jeopardize underlying bony tissue to devitalization. The goal of oral soft tissue treatment is to reestablish vital soft tissue bony coverage.

Abrasion

Abrasion is a superficial wound, which is likened to a surface rub or wear of the epithelial or gingival tissue. Treatment basically consists of local cleansing with a disinfectant soap for the skin and saline or 0.12% chlorhexidine irrigation for the gingiva. Always closely inspect the wound for foreign body insult, which is associated with accidental gingival tattooing.

Contusion

Contusion results from trauma that produces hemorrhage of subcutaneous tissue without a break of the overlying soft tissue, similar to a bruising injury or an underlying hematoma formation. Treatment involves local cleansing and observation, essentially self-limiting.

Laceration

Lacertion is the separation of the superficial tissue layer. It should be considered in a linear or complex grouping and may

Table 2	Treatment of pediatric injuries
Type of Injury	Treatment
Crown Fractures	
Class I (enamel only)	Smooth rough edges
Class II (enamel and dentin)	1. CaOH or class ionomer liner over dentin
	2. Composite resin restoration
Class III (Pulpal Involvement)	
Vital pulp	1. Formocresol pulpotomy
	2. Coronal coverage
Nonvital pulp	1. ZnOH-eugenol pulpectomy
	2. Coronal coverage
Class IV (Root Fractures)	
Apical 3rd	No treatment; follow-up
Cervical 3rd	1. Remove tooth fragments
	2. Allow apical 3rd to resorb if compromise to permanent tooth bud is expected
Luxations	
Subluxation	Monitor/follow-up
Lateral luxations	Realign/remove as needed
Extrusion	Realign/remove as needed
Intrusion	1. Allow to reerupt 4–6 wk
	2. Remove if in contact with permanent successor
	3. Remove if infection presents

be associated with an underlying bony defect. Treatment involves thorough cleansing, reapproximation, and stabilization with sutures. If necessary, devitalized tissue is judiciously excised in a conservative manner. Consider antibiotic and tetanus prophylaxis.

Pediatric dentoalveolar trauma treatment

In the pediatric population, poor coordination resulting in falls is the primary cause of dentoalveolar trauma injuries. From a dental standpoint, the large pulp chamber/tooth ratio also expounds on this class of injuries. Displacements are more prevalent than tooth fractures because of the relative resilience of the surrounding bone. Treatment is based on the likelihood that the permanent tooth bud may be compromised, secondary to the buccal-occlusal position of the primary teeth

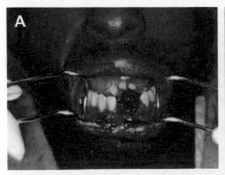
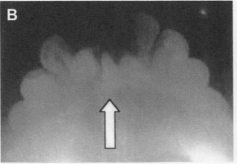
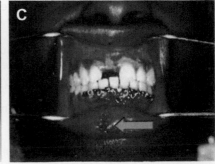

Fig. 20 (A) Blunt facial trauma resulting in alveolar fracture and perioral soft tissue lacerations. (B) Occlusal radiograph confirms alveolar fracture with lingual displacement (apical lock) of mandibular central incisors and left incisors (arrow). (C) Alveolar fracture disimpaction, reduction, and stabilization with arch wire. Debridement and repair of perioral soft tissue (arrow).

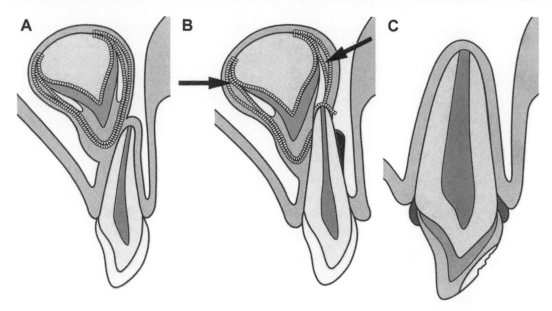

Fig. 21 (*A*) Normal position of primary tooth to permanent tooth bud. (*B*) Apical intrusion of primary root impinging on permanent tooth bud. *Blue arrows* denote permanent tooth bud. (*C*) Hypoplasia of permanent tooth secondary to apical intrusion.

to the permanent tooth bud. The general treatment of pediatric dental injuries is summarized in Table 2.

Andreasen and Ravn[15] reported on the general prognosis of the traumatized permanent successors, secondary to forces applied by the primary dentition. They found that the individual's age at the time of injury and the type of luxation play a major role in the errant development of the permanent dentition (Fig. 21).

References

1. Shayne's dental site. History of dentistry, Greco-Roman dentistry (AD 350–750), Available at: http://www.dental-site.itgo.com/grecoroman.htm. Accessed March 17, 2003.
2. Lockhart PB, Feldbau EV, Gabel RA, et al. Dental complications during and after tracheal intubation. J Am Dent Assoc 1986;112:480.
3. Wright RB, Mansfield FF. Damage to teeth during the administration of general anesthesia. Anesth Analg 1974;53:450.
4. Piercell MP, White DE, Nelson R. Prevention of self-inflicted trauma in semicomatose patients. J Oral Surg 1974;32:903.
5. Andreasen JO. Classification, etiology and epidemiology. In: Andreases JO, editor. Traumatic injuries of the teeth. 2nd edition. Copenhagen (Denmark): Munksgaard; 1981. p. 19.
6. Davidoff G, Jakubowski M, Thomas D, et al. The spectrum of closed-head injury in facial trauma victims: incidence and impact. Ann Emerg Med 1988;17:27.
7. Bucci MN, Phillips TJ, McGillicuddy JE. Delayed epidural hemorrhage in hypotensive multiple trauma patients. Neurosurgery 1986; 19:65–8.
8. Fulling H-J, Andreasen JO. Influence of maturation status and tooth type of permanent teeth upon electrometric and thermal pulp testing. Scand J Dent Res 1976;84:286–90.
9. John son DJ. Innervation of teeth: qualitative, quantitative, and developmental assessment. J Dent Res 1985;64:555–63.
10. Andreasen JO, Andreasen FM. Textbook and color atlas of traumatic injuries to the teeth. 3rd edition. Copenhagen (Denmark): Munksgaard; 1994. p. 202–10, 315–77, 383.
11. Andreasen JO. Luxation of permanent teeth due to trauma: a clinical and radiographic follow-up study of 189 injured teeth. Scand J Dent Res 1970;78:273.
12. Andreasen JO, Sundstrom B, Ravn JJ. The effect of traumatic injuries to primary teeth on their permanent successors. I. A clinical, radiographic, microradiographic and electronmicroscopic study of 117 injured permanent teeth. Scand J Dent Res 1970;79:219–83.
13. Andreasen JO, Ravn JJ. The effect of traumatic injuries to primary teeth on their permanent successors. II. A clinical and radiographic follow-up of 213 injured teeth. Scand J Dent Res 1970;79: 284–94.
14. Andreasen FM, Vestergaard Pedersen B. Prognosis of luxated permanent teeth—the development of pulp necrosis. Endod Dent Traumatol 1985;1:207–20.
15. Lieblich SE. Surgical aspects of apicoectomy with "hands on" demonstration of microapical preparation. Surgical minilectures (M222). J Oral Maxillofac Surg 2003;100.

Evidence-Based Surgical-Orthodontic Management of Impacted Teeth

Keith Sherwood, DDS [a,b,*]

KEYWORDS

- Canines • Eruption • Orthodontics • Exposure • Bracketing

KEY POINTS

- Other than third molars, the maxillary canine teeth are the most commonly impacted teeth.
- Surgical intervention and coordination of care with the orthodontist will lead to improved outcomes.
- Various surgical procedures are used depending on the position of the impacted tooth.

Introduction

Interdisciplinary management of impacted teeth represents one of the most important cooperative interactions between oral and maxillofacial surgeons and orthodontists. Most patients requiring exposure of an impacted tooth are referred for surgery by an orthodontist. The diagnostic work is usually assumed by the orthodontist, who will have treatment preferences and abilities based on training and experience. The orthodontist often is dissociated from surgical planning or, conversely, may request inappropriate treatment. By contrast, surgeons usually learn a generic surgical approach for orthodontically managed impactions, and may receive an incomplete didactic background in diagnosis and treatment planning. Orthodontic mechanics are largely opaque to surgeons, and this puts them at a disadvantage in helping to individualize the surgical plan for their comanaged patient. This division of labor, though valuable, can negatively affect the speed and success of postoperative orthodontics.

The purpose of this report is to provide an evidence-based approach for the treatment of impacted teeth that require joint orthodontic and surgical care. Although the focus is on the management of ectopic canines, the principles can be applied to any impacted tooth that needs alignment. This approach is designed to facilitate communication between the oral and maxillofacial surgeon and the orthodontist, and improve the predictability, ease, and success of treatment.

Incidence and etiology

Studies reporting the incidence of impacted teeth vary considerably in their conclusions, likely due to regional genetic differences, the dental health of the population studied, and interpretation of what constitutes impaction.

Aside from third molars, maxillary canines are the most commonly impacted teeth.[1,2] There is a 2:1 incidence among females over males and a 2 to 3 times higher likelihood of palatal versus labial impaction.[3] The incidence of maxillary impaction has been reported to be between 1% and 5% in different populations. A lower frequency has been noted among Blacks and Asians[4] and there is a higher occurrence in Greeks and Turks,[5,6] with European Caucasians somewhere in between.[3,7] Reports of rates as high as 23.5% may occur in individual orthodontic practices.[8] Even if we assume a 1% to 2% incidence, the number of patients affected is enormous. As pointed out by Dewel,[9] the canine has the longest, most complex eruption path as well as the slowest development time. It should perhaps be no surprise that it is often impacted.

The etiology of impacted canines, especially palatally displaced teeth, is speculative. There are 2 major theories reported extensively in the literature. The genetic theory suggests that impactions are primarily caused by gene mediation, probably polygenic multifactorial inheritance.[10] Although genetic mechanisms are difficult to prove, the presence of familial similarities, gender differences, and the acceptance of gene mechanisms with other dental anomalies argue strongly for a genetic connection.

Alternatively the guidance theory proposes an environmental factor, specifically the lack of normal contact between the lateral incisor root and the erupting canine.[11] It is well known that anomalous and missing lateral incisors are often seen with palatally impacted canines. Furthermore, there is little argument that environmental factors such as crowding, irradiation, endocrine disorders, gingival scarring, and trauma all may cause impacted canines.

It is likely that both genetics and environmental factors cause impacted teeth. However, diagnosis and treatment success in managing impacted canines, as with other health problems, can be strongly influenced by a better understanding of etiology.

Early diagnosis

After the age of 9 or 10 years when patients often first consult with the orthodontist, there are well-established warning signs of potential canine impaction.[12]

Disclosures: The author has nothing to disclose.
[a] Department of Orthodontics, Goldman School of Dental Medicine, Boston University, 100 E. Newton Street, Boston, MA 02118, USA
[b] Department of Oral and Maxillofacial Surgery, Beverly Hospital, 85 Herrick Street, Beverly, MA 01915, USA
* 80 Lindall Street, Hunt Medical Building, Suite #4, Danvers, MA 01923.
E-mail address: ksomsortho@yahoo.com

Atlas Oral Maxillofacial Surg Clin N Am 21 (2013) 199–210
1061-3315/13/$ - see front matter © 2013 Elsevier Inc. All rights reserved.
http://dx.doi.org/10.1016/j.cxom.2013.05.006

Clinical signs include:
- Absence of the canine bulge with palatal impactions (Fig. 1)
- Peg-shaped or missing lateral incisors
- A constricted maxilla with dental crowding
- Female patients 2:1 higher incidence
- Class I occlusion in the mixed dentition

Radiographic signs include (Fig. 2)[13]:
- Lateral or central incisor overlapped by the erupting canine
- Enlarged follicular sac of the erupting canine
- Lack of resorption of the root of the primary canine
- Presence of impacted mandibular bicuspids[14,15]

Sajnani and King[16] have developed an early radiographic prediction of impaction based on angulation of the erupting canine to the midline and distance from the occlusal plane on panographs.

Early diagnosis and treatment of canine displacement avoids the potentially serious risk of resorption of incisor roots (Fig. 3). This injury is common, can begin in the early stages of impaction,[17] and may lead to loss of teeth. Retained impacted teeth may eventually cause arch-length discrepancies, ankylosis, compromised orthodontic treatment, and the potential development of significant disorder.

Clinical management of the impacted canine

Interceptive treatment

Interceptive treatment may reduce the incidence or severity of canine impactions. Although inconclusive, some studies have shown an improved spontaneous eruption of developmentally delayed canines when the primary canine is extracted.[18] It is not fully understood why this strategy expedites canine eruption, although removing an obstacle to eruption is the prevailing orthodontic rationale. However, the "Regional Acceleratory Phenomena"[19,20,35] may be an underlying contributory factor. This theory, which has gained traction in the orthodontic community, maintains that bone trauma results in physiologic bone remodeling (in this case from the extraction), which can indirectly facilitate regional tooth movement.

Other studies have shown improvement in canine displacement with orthodontic interventions such as palatal expanders,

headgear, and distalization mechanics.[21] The success of such orthodontic approaches lend support to the guidance theory or local environment effect on the etiology of canine impaction as discussed earlier.

Surgical management of the impacted canine

Treatment planning for impacted canines is based on an understanding of the etiology. Selection of surgical technique, however, is driven by the location of the affected tooth, the needs of the orthodontist, periodontal concerns, and individual patient factors. As with orthognathic surgery, good communication between the orthodontist and surgeon is critical to successful and efficient treatment.

There are 2 general approaches to the surgical treatment of ectopic canines. Closed-flap forced eruption, whereby the gingival flap is sutured back over the canine after exposure and bracketing, and open exposure, with or without packing or bracketing, to create an epithelialized fenestration or window through the gingiva that leaves the canine visible. Many studies and opinion pieces have been reported supporting one particular surgical approach over another. However, each method offers specific advantages and disadvantages that clinicians should understand, to help in treatment planning and obtaining improved clinical results.

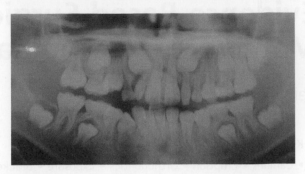

Fig. 2 Radiograph of signs of canine impaction. Peg laterals, overlap lateral roots, retained primary canines, and enlarged follicular sacs.

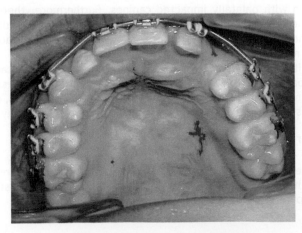

Fig. 1 Lack of canine bulge.

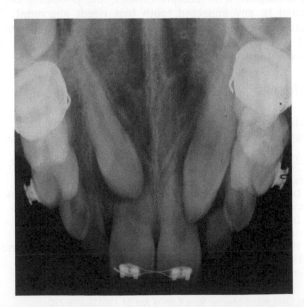

Fig. 3 Root resorption central incisors from impacted canines.

The accepted surgical techniques are outlined here. These methods are discussed and compared more in depth in the following sections, including indications, advantages and disadvantages, orthodontic and surgical preparation, evidence base for decision making, and case reports.

- Closed-flap forced eruption: labial or palatal impactions
- Open passive eruption
  - Labial: apically positioned flap
  - Palatal: open packing technique
- Open exposure, forced eruption

Closed-flap forced eruption

The closed-flap forced eruption technique is one of the most popular and versatile surgical approaches for canine impaction management (Figs. 4–7).

A gingival crevicular incision is made palatally or labially, and a full-thickness mucoperiosteal envelope flap is elevated over the impacted tooth. The length of the incision is related to the depth of impaction. Palatally, the incision will typically extend at least 2 teeth on either side of the impaction site (see Figs. 4 and 5). Division of the incisal nerve on the palate is usually unnecessary. Bone is removed where necessary, and a bracket attached to a gold chain or wire is cemented onto the buccal or lingual of the impacted tooth (see Figs. 6 and 7). Most studies recommend avoiding excessive bone removal, which may lead to periodontal defects and gingival recession. Of particular concern is bone removal apical to the cementoenamel junction.[22,23] With palatal impactions, some clinicians will remove a channel of bone between the root socket of the extracted primary canine and the crown of the impacted canine (Fig. 8). Although designed to expedite eruption, and intuitively attractive, there are no data to either support or refute this practice. However, because orthodontic tooth movement through bone is a slow physiologic process of resorption and remodeling, the value of additional bone removal still needs to be researched before it can be recommended.

The orthodontic bracket can be cemented only after good exposure and moisture control. Extra cement will help resist debonding (for bracketing tips, see the technical section). The flap is closed primarily, and the chain or wire attached to the bracket exits the wound through the incision and is tied to the arch wire. The orthodontist uses the chain or wire to attach springs or elastic thread, which erupts the impacted tooth. Appropriate forces are necessary because excessive orthodontic

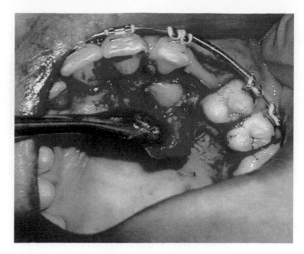

Fig. 5   Elevated flap.

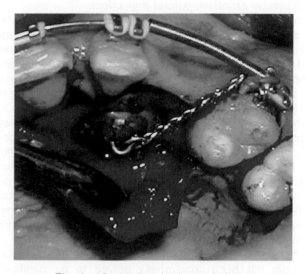

Fig. 6   Canine bracketing and chain.

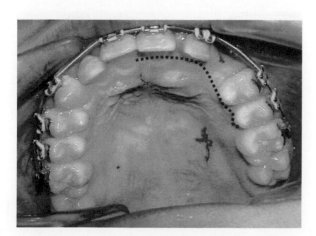

Fig. 4   Outline of incision line for palatal flap.

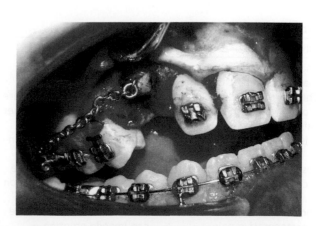

Fig. 7   Labial envelope flap, canine bracketing.

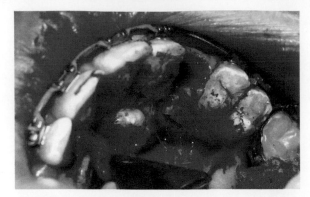

Fig. 8 Bone excision between primary canine socket and impacted canine (*arrows*).

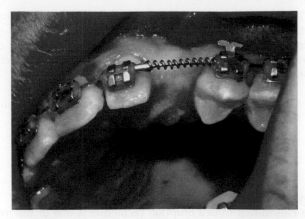

Fig. 9 Thick palatal gingiva and lack of bulge.

force will actually slow or stop eruption of the treated tooth owing to hyalinization of the periodontal ligament.

The advantages and disadvantages of a closed-flap forced eruption are summarized in Table 1.

Open passive eruption

Open passive eruption, palatal impactions

Open passive eruption requires a fenestration made through the gingiva, and the impacted tooth is allowed to erupt spontaneously through the opening (Figs. 9–14). It is a time-honored approach that has been in use since before adequate composite cements were available for orthodontic bracketing. The theory that the presence of a thick gingival covering (see Fig. 9) slows the natural eruption process is appealing because of the observation that gingival fibrosis can lead to delayed eruption.[26] In addition, gingival tissue is flexible and expandable, due in part to the presence histologically of elastic fibers (see Fig. 10). It is not known whether the ability of soft tissue to accommodate pressure and expand without breaking open during the eruption process helps to keep an erupting tooth confined. However, this is often the premise when exposing an impacted tooth (with or without bone removal) and allowing it to erupt spontaneously.

The speed of eruption and completion of the orthodontic case has not been conclusively proved to be significantly affected by whether a closed forced eruption or an open passive eruption technique has been used to treat the palatally impacted canine.[27] Unfortunately, most studies are either retrospective or have a limited number of subjects. Nearly all are adversely affected by the lack of control of variables such

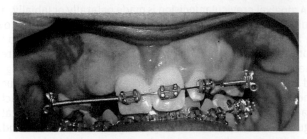

Fig. 10 Tenting of stretched gingiva over impacted canine.

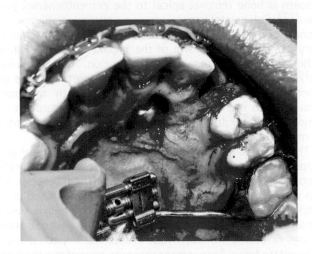

Fig. 11 Palatal window through flap after canine exposure.

Table 1 Closed-flap forced eruption	
Advantages	Disadvantages
The impacted tooth can be aligned while it is erupted	Cannot see erupting tooth without a radiograph
There are no packings or open wounds	If bracket debonds it requires another surgery to rebracket
Labial attached gingiva is maintained[24]	May take longer to erupt canine compared with open forced eruption
Less scarring and periodontal concerns[25]	Orthodontists prefer to see tooth during forced-eruption process to help align
For palatal impactions, less postoperative pain	Excessive orthodontic force can impede eruption

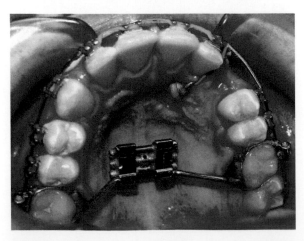

Fig. 12 Delayed bracketing at 8 weeks after surgery.

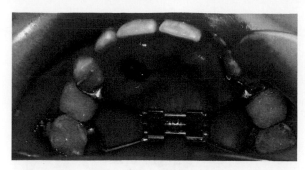

Fig. 13 Open exposure, 1 week after surgery.

Table 2 Open, passive eruption

Advantages and indications	Disadvantages
Advantageous for impacted teeth that are not too deeply embedded in bone or acutely angled	More painful for patient
Can be used with or without orthodontic appliances but bracketing often easier 2–4 wk postoperative in a dry field	Requires multiple packing changes
Allows visualization of tooth for orthodontic control	Not ideal for teeth deeply embedded in bone or severely angled

as orthodontic eruption mechanics, depth of impaction, tooth angulation, and patient age, all of which have been shown to affect time of treatment and prognosis.[28]

The surgical technique is identical to the flap elevation with closed eruption, but a fenestration or window is made through the palatal gingiva over the affected canine (see Fig. 11). The window must be large enough to expose most of one surface of the crown of the impacted tooth to account for the inevitable regrowth of the gingiva. The flap is sutured back in place and a packing inserted into the wound. The favored packing material is usually 0.25-inch (0.64-cm) gauze strip often impregnated with an antimicrobial or anesthetizing paste. The packing is sutured in place for 7 to 10 days. After preliminary healing the packing should be changed weekly until adequate eruption occurs for true passive eruption, or a bracket can be applied to the tooth when possible and forced eruption instituted (see Figs. 12–14).

Though dated, the open packing technique is still favored by some surgeons and orthodontists as either a primary technique or an interim step before bracketing. For the surgeon it has the virtue of shifting the responsibility for bracketing back to the orthodontist, who has more experience with the procedure. For the orthodontist it allows visualization of the impacted tooth, and can be a very effective technique for spontaneous eruption. It has largely been displaced by the closed technique in popularity, especially with deeply impacted teeth, because of the nuisance of changing packings for the clinician and patient, and lack of control of the eruption vector. There is also more discomfort for the patient owing to the fenestration.

Table 2 lists the indications, advantages, and disadvantages of the open passive eruption technique.

Apically positioned flap for labial impactions
The apically positioned flap (APF) has long been used for periodontally compromised patients to reduce buccal

pocketing and improve access for hygiene (Figs. 15–20). Vanarsdall and Corn[22] reported extensively on the importance of erupting the canine into attached gingiva to prevent thinning of this zone and recession. The APF properly applied to the exposure of impacted canines uniquely prevents this complication. It can be used effectively as a passive eruption technique or, more commonly, for open forced eruption by cementing a bracket immediately or after preliminary healing.

As shown in Figs. 15–20, the procedure involves placing vertical labial-releasing incisions mesial and distal to the impacted tooth from the gingival crest to just below the margin of the attached and unattached gingiva, and slightly farther apart than the estimated width of the canine (see Fig. 15). A crestal incision connecting the vertical cuts should fall short of contact with the adjacent teeth, avoiding the papilla. A full-thickness flap is developed and retracted apically. More apical retraction is possible with longer-releasing incisions and periosteum release. Enough of the thin labial bone is removed, and the soft tissue apically positioned to allow partial exposure of the labial enamel crown surface, and if desired, placement of an orthodontic attachment (see Figs. 16–20). A bonded bracket will help to stabilize the flap during healing.

The retracted crestal gingival tissue is managed based on the need for adding labial attached gingiva. The goal should be a healthy band of attached gingiva that slightly exceeds the vertical width of tissue on the contralateral side. If more attached labial gingiva is required, some of the crestal gingiva at the flap margin is sutured more apical to the exposed labial crown surface. If there is adequate labial attached gingiva preoperatively, the surplus retracted crestal tissue can be excised as needed. Palatal gingiva can also be excised if necessary.

Care must be taken with the APF to avoid the gingival papilla in flap development to prevent blunting of the papillae and embrasure defects. Gentle tissue manipulation is important to reduce scarring.

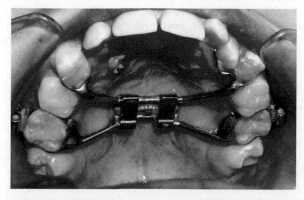

Fig. 14 Delayed bracketing at 4 weeks after surgery.

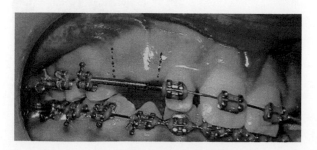

Fig. 15 Outline of apically positioned flap.

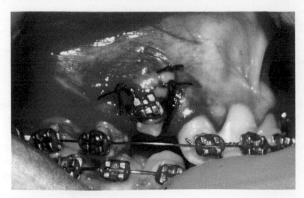

Fig. 16 Apically positioned flap. Standard bracket used to stabilize flap.

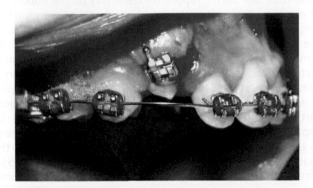

Fig. 17 Healing and passive eruption 1 week after surgery.

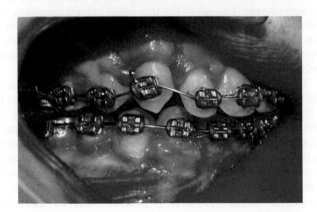

Fig. 18 Passive eruption at 2 months after surgery. Bracket engaged. Note excellent band of attached gingiva.

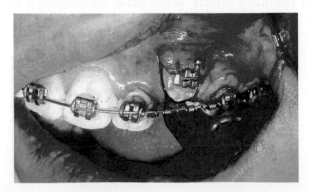

Fig. 19 Apically positioned flap, and flap-stabilizing bracket.

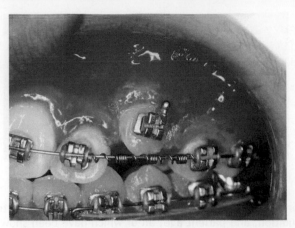

Fig. 20 Passive eruption at 1 month after surgery.

Many orthodontists prefer the APF for labial canine exposure because it allows visualization of the impacted tooth and seems to speed eruption. However, if the tooth is too deeply impacted it is an impractical procedure. Vermette and colleagues[25] have reported more cosmetic and periodontal issues than are encountered with the envelope flap.

The advantages and disadvantages of the APF for open passive eruption are outlined in Table 3.

Open exposure, forced eruption

Combining open exposure with forced eruption labially (Figs. 21–23), or palatally (Figs. 24–28), when possible, is often favored by orthodontists because of the perception that the impacted tooth can be erupted and aligned more quickly and safely. Providing visibility of the treated canine prevents it from putting excess pressure on the roots of adjacent teeth, which can lead to root resorption or stop the eruption process. Removing overlying gingiva reduces the potential contribution of gingival restraint on the erupting tooth.

The technique is similar to open passive eruption surgery, but includes placement of a bracket for immediate orthodontic traction. Less gingiva is removed, and flaps are less extensive and sutured back enough to allow just partial visibility of the tooth and bracket.

There are no definitive studies that compare the speed of treatment between open exposure, forced eruption of impacted canines, and other techniques. Indeed, most of the reports discussing speed of treatment examine open passive versus closed forced eruption of palatal canines.[3,27,29,30] However, many experienced orthodontists believe that bracketing the canine at the time of surgery or soon after, and guiding it into its appropriate position in the arch, more effectively and quickly treats the displacement. Furthermore, if we are to accept the notion that soft tissue restricts tooth eruption, the combination

Table 3 Apically positioned flap

Advantages	Disadvantages
Indicated especially when there is a need to widen or preserve the zone of attached gingiva	If done injudiciously, may result in more cosmetic and periodontal concerns
Allows visualization of impacted tooth	Not suitable for more deeply impacted teeth
May expedite eruption	Technique sensitive

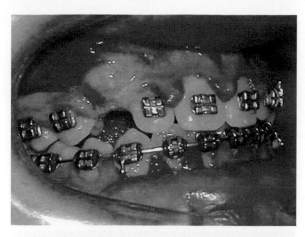

Fig. 21 Preoperative combined open-closed eruption technique with apically positioned flap.

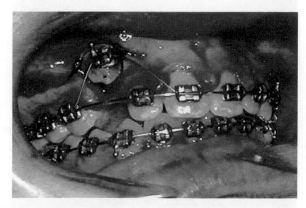

Fig. 22 Combined open-closed exposure, apically positioned flap, forced eruption with superelastic nickel-titanium wire.

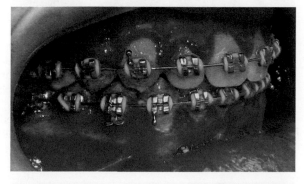

Fig. 23 Combined open-closed eruption with full alignment at 8 weeks after surgery.

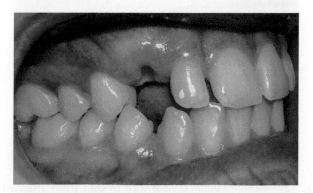

Fig. 24 Sixteen-year-old palatally impacted canines.

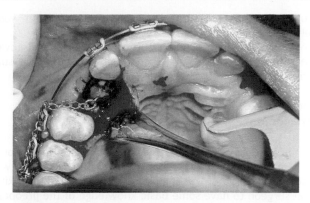

Fig. 25 Palatal flap for combined open-closed exposure for forced eruption.

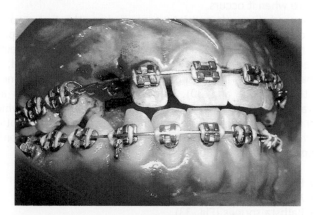

Fig. 26 Flap closure with crestal gingiva excised, partial exposure of bracket, and incisal edge of canine.

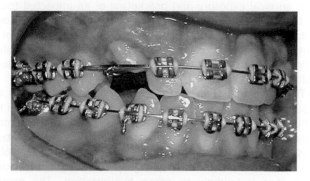

Fig. 27 Three weeks after surgery: forced eruption and emergence of incisal edge.

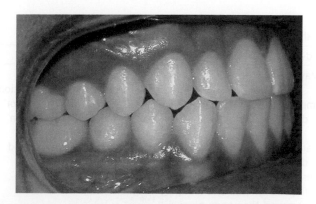

Fig. 28 Full alignment at 12 weeks after combined-exposure forced eruption.

of open exposure with judicious orthodontic traction would likely speed canine alignment.

With these points in mind, the advantages and disadvantages of the open exposure forced eruption option are summarized in Table 4.

Preoperative and postsurgical orthodontic management

It is not within the scope of this article to detail orthodontic mechanics in treating ectopic canines. However, as with orthognathic surgery, it is important for the oral and maxillofacial surgeon to have some basic knowledge of the preoperative and postsurgical orthodontics to facilitate communication and treatment, and to be in a position to objectively evaluate failure when it occurs.

Beyond diagnosis and interceptive care, the first step for the orthodontist is usually to evaluate the available arch space for the erupting canine. If the primary canine is lost prematurely, as is often the case, and arch space is diminished, an expansion coil spring is used to create room for the permanent tooth (Figs. 29 and 30). The orthodontic arch wires are advanced over time to a heavy rectangular steel wire, which can resist deformation and act as a stable anchor for eruption springs, wires, or elastic thread. Commonly used orthodontic eruption devices include:

- Elastic thread (Fig. 31)
- Auxiliary, superelastic nickel-titanium wire (Fig. 32)
- Ballista springs (Fig. 33)

There are 2 major orthodontic causes of retarded eruption after surgical exposure and bracketing of an impacted tooth: contact of the canine crown with an adjacent immobile tooth root, and excessive orthodontic force placed on the erupting canine. Undue orthodontic force on a tooth leads to hyalinization of the periodontal ligament, arrested tooth movement, and, possibly, ankylosis.

The challenge then for the orthodontist is to move the impacted canine around the roots of adjacent teeth with the right amount of force. Ballista springs, for example, will move a palatally impacted tooth lingually away from the lateral incisor root. Extrusive forces on a tooth should not exceed 60 g. Nickel-titanium wires and springs provide light continuous force that is unlikely to cause hyalinization. The popular elastic thread is quick and easy to use, but determining force levels with this method is difficult. The eruption process can

Table 4 Open-exposure forced eruption

Advantages	Disadvantages
May result in speedier eruption	Excessive orthodontic force can impede eruption
Impacted tooth is visible during eruption	May result in cosmetic or periodontal problems on the labia
Can be used with moderately deep impactions	More painful than closed eruption
Less flap elevation than closed flap technique, and less gingiva removed than open passive procedure	

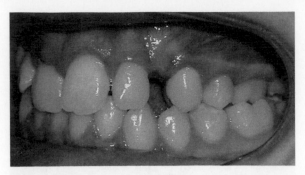

Fig. 29   Loss of space for canine.

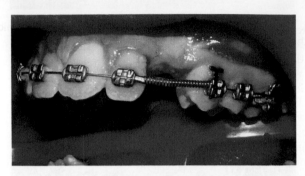

Fig. 30   Open coil spring to create interdental space for erupting canine.

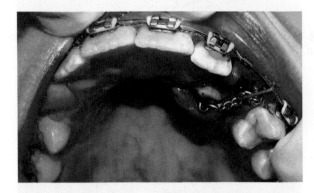

Fig. 31   Elastic thread, combined open-closed eruption.

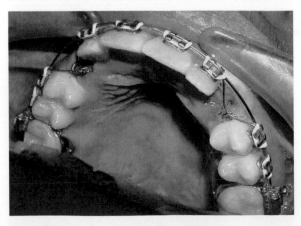

Fig. 32   Nickel-titanium double wire to gold chain attached to impacted canines open-closed forced eruption.

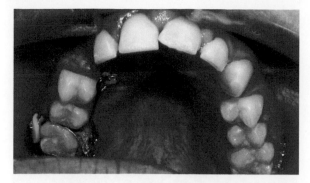

Fig. 33 Ballista spring for closed eruption.

take anywhere from a few weeks to more than a year, depending on the location of the impacted tooth and the skill of the orthodontist.

When the closed forced eruption technique is used, the orthodontist must often guess at the location and orientation of the impacted tooth based on radiographs. In the postoperative report to the orthodontist, the surgeon should detail the axial position of the impacted tooth and its contact with adjacent roots. A photo can be a valuable aid for an orthodontic colleague and a practice builder.

Technical tips for the surgeon to prevent surgically related problems

1. Preparation for surgery begins with localization of the impacted canine. As reported by Becker, an inaccurate understanding of the location of the ectopic tooth is a major contributing factor in failure or inefficiency of treatment, for both the surgeon and orthodontist.[31] The combination of an astute clinical examination and radiographic analysis will reliably locate the canine and avoid unnecessary surgery. The absence of the canine bulge suggests a palatal impaction. A buccal or lingual bulge or asymmetry in palpation of cortical contours will also help with location.

    Good 3-dimensional radiographic analysis of the position of the impacted tooth is required, especially for palatal impactions.[32] Although cone-beam computed tomography imaging can provide specific information, standard periapical radiographs using the Clark buccal slide rule, or an occlusal film and panograph using the vertical parallax rule, may be adequate and result in less radiation exposure (Figs. 34 and 35).

2. Bracketing can be a source of concern for the surgeon. Debonding of the bracket during closed eruption is a significant complication for the surgeon, orthodontist, and patient. Surgery must be redone, orthodontic treatment will be prolonged for months, and the patient suffers. Blood and saliva contamination is the major cause of debonding from the tooth surface. However, brackets can separate from the cement as well. Some tips on bracketing to eliminate debonding problems are listed here.
    - Good exposure of the impacted tooth and retraction of the soft tissues go a long way toward avoiding contamination of enamel surface.
    - Use of hydrogen peroxide on a cotton-tip applicator to clean the tooth will remove surface film and blood. Some clinicians apply acid etch, which accomplishes the same

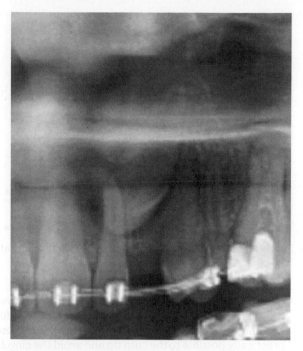

Fig. 34 Pan view showing canine overlapping lateral at mid-root.

goal but may cause tissue necrosis. These substances must be rinsed off well before bracketing.
    - The use of a self-etching, moisture-resistant, light-cured bonding agent and cement will reduce bond failure.
    - Bracket placement will affect eruption speed. Basic biomechanics dictates that the closer the bracket is to the incisal edge of the tooth, the easier and quicker it is for the

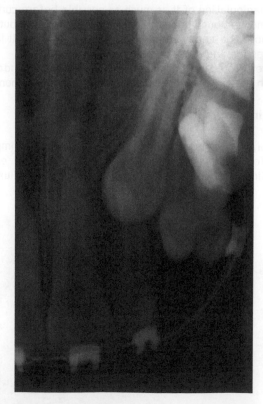

Fig. 35 Parallax principle. Occlusal view, showing palatal canine moving apical to more labial lateral incisor.

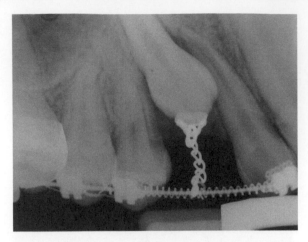

Fig. 36   Ideal bracket placement to allow rapid cuspid rotation.

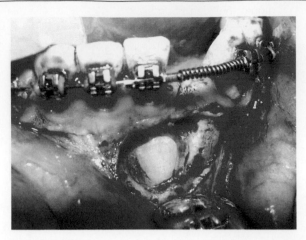

Fig. 38   Corticotomy around ankylosed tooth after failed forced eruption.

orthodontist to rotate it to the proper position (Fig. 36); this is especially true for steeply angled teeth. However, the bracket requires a relatively flat surface during cementation for stability. Bracket the canine as close as practically possible to the cusp tip and avoid the cingulum.

- There are 2 strategies to prevent the bracket from separating from the cement: (1) place a small dab of the primer on the mesh of the bracket with the sponge stick before adding cement; (2) after initial bracket placement and curing, consider adding an increment of cement over the bracket margins with an explorer tip and the sponge stick from the primer (Fig. 37).
- The button bracket is the most adaptable for lingual bracketing. A chain with extra-large links is easier for the orthodontist to use.
- Once the bracket has been applied, avoid further manipulation of it as much as possible before curing.

3. Remove enough bone to allow a clean, dry field but never expose the cementoenamel junction, as this will lead to recession and other periodontal problems.

4. Careful soft-tissue manipulation and cosmetic wound closure with the APF reduces scarring and wound contraction.

Managing complications

The major complications related to exposure of impacted teeth for orthodontic manipulation are failure to erupt,[33] debonding, and cosmetic or periodontal issues. A "luxation"

may be requested by the orthodontist. Though reported anecdotally, the value of subluxation is debatable. There are no good studies supporting this technique, and serious risks of pulpal necrosis, external root resorption, bone loss, and true ankylosis as seen with traumatized teeth are possible. It should be considered only as a last resort, and only with teeth with an open apex and less than 75% root development.[34] Instead, an organized and more measured protocol may salvage the case.

1. Managing forced-eruption failure
   - Diagnosis. The first sign that the impacted canine is not erupting is the development of an open bite. The canine acts as an anchor and intrudes the adjacent teeth instead of erupting.
   - Orthodontist responsibility. The orthodontist should be aware of this and stop all forces on the canine for a month. Lighter forces can then begin. If there is likely contact with an adjacent root (ie, the lateral incisor) the affected tooth should be debracketed to allow it to move out of the way as the canine erupts.
   - Surgeon's responsibility. If these orthodontic steps fail, additional surgery will be needed. If forced closed eruption was attempted the first time, consider an open packing, passive eruption technique. According to some reports, combining this with corticotomy of the adjacent bone may facilitate tooth movement by triggering the regional acceleratory phenomenon (Fig. 38).[35] When

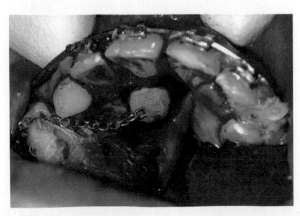

Fig. 37   Extra cement added to bracket margins.

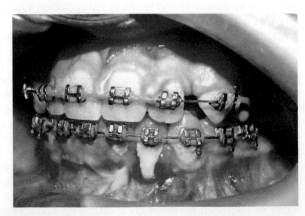

Fig. 39   Residual periodontal defect caused by loss of bone during forced eruption.

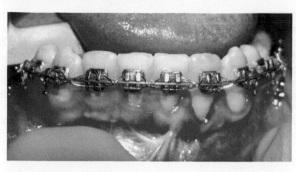

Fig. 40 Root coverage after bone grafting, membrane, and bipedicled flap repair.

orthodontic force is restarted on the tooth, it should be very light.

2. Preventing debonding has been discussed in the previous section on technical tips. If rebonding is necessary, consider an open packing procedure with delayed bracketing for the next surgery. If a closed procedure is preferred, thoroughly remove any retained cement from the tooth, re-etch, and follow the aforesaid recommendations for bracketing.

3. Cosmetic and periodontal complications are largely preventable with careful management of hard and soft tissue. However, with extensive labial bone loss from surgery or orthodontics, significant gingival recession is an unsightly complication that can be improved with bone grafting and gingival rotation flaps. Some surgeons defer this treatment to a periodontist, although the procedures are fairly straightforward. Plastic principles of gentle tissue manipulation and tension-free closure are critical (Figs. 39 and 40).

Summary

Ideal management of the impacted canine is a complex process involving a carefully orchestrated effort on the part of the orthodontist, surgeon, and others. Communication among clinicians is an essential component of successful treatment. This communication should include which type of surgical approach is to be used for the specific case. The surgeon needs to understand the various treatment options.

Evidence-based diagnosis, treatment planning, and appropriate technique can result in a highly successful and gratifying outcome.

References

1. McSherry P. The assessment of and treatment options for the buried maxillary canine. Dent Update 1996;23(1):7–10.
2. Shafer WG, Hine MK, Levy BM. Textbook of oral pathology. St. Louis, MO: W.B Saunders Company; 1974.
3. Bishara SE. Impacted maxillary canines: a review. Am J Orthod Dentofacial Orthop 1992;101(2):159–71.
4. Kramer RM, Williams AC. The incidence of impacted teeth. A survey at Harlem hospital. Oral Surg Oral Med Oral Pathol 1970;29(2):237–41.
5. Fardi A, Kondylidou-Sidira A, Bachour Z, et al. Incidence of impacted and supernumerary teeth-a radiographic study in a North Greek population. Med Oral Patol Oral Cir Bucal 2011;16(1):e56–61.
6. Aydin U, Yilmaz HH, Yildirim D. Incidence of canine impaction and transmigration in a patient population. Dentomaxillofac Radiol 2004;33:164–9.
7. Thilander B, Myrberg N. The prevalence of malocclusion in Swedish schoolchildren. Scand J Dent Res 1973;81(1):12–21.
8. Ferguson JW, Pitt SK. Management of unerupted maxillary canines where no orthodontic treatment is planned; a survey of UK consultant opinion. J Orthod 2004;31(1):28–33.
9. Dewel BF. Clinical observations on the axial inclination of teeth. Am J Orthod 1949;35(2):98–115.
10. Peck S, Peck L, Kataja M. The palatally displaced canine as a dental anomaly of genetic origin. Angle Orthod 1994;64(4):249–56.
11. Becker A. In defense of the guidance theory of palatal canine displacement. Angle Orthod 1995;65(2):95–8.
12. Ericson S, Kurol J. Longitudinal study and analysis of clinical supervision of maxillary canine eruption. Community Dent Oral Epidemiol 1986;14(3):172–6.
13. Ericson S, Kurol J. Radiographic examination of ectopically erupting maxillary canines. Am J Orthod Dentofacial Orthop 1987;91(6):483–92.
14. Baccetti T, Leonardi M, Giuntini V. Distally displaced premolars: a dental anomaly associated with palatally displaced canines. Am J Orthod Dentofacial Orthop 2010;138(3):318–22.
15. Garib DG, Alencar BM, Lauris JR, et al. Agenesis of maxillary lateral incisors and associated dental anomalies. Am J Orthod Dentofacial Orthop 2010;137(6):732.e1–6.
16. Sajnani AK, King NM. Early prediction of maxillary canine impaction from panoramic radiographs. Am J Orthod Dentofacial Orthop 2012;142(1):45–51.
17. Ericson S, Kurol J. Resorption of maxillary lateral incisors caused by ectopic eruption of the canines. A clinical and radiographic analysis of predisposing factors. Am J Orthod Dentofacial Orthop 1988;94(6):503–13.
18. Jacobs SG. Reducing the incidence of unerupted palatally displaced canines by extraction of deciduous canines. The history and application of this procedure with some case reports. Aust Dent J 1998;43(1):20–7.
19. Strippoli J, Aknin JJ. Accelerated tooth movement by alveolar corticotomy or piezocision. Orthod Fr 2012;83(2):155–64 [in French].
20. Mostafa YA, Mohamed Salah Fayed M, Mehanni S, et al. Comparison of corticotomy-facilitated vs standard tooth-movement techniques in dogs with miniscrews as anchor units. Am J Orthod Dentofacial Orthop 2009;136(4):570–7.
21. Baccetti T, Mucedero M, Leonardi M, et al. Interceptive treatment of palatal impaction of maxillary canines with rapid maxillary expansion: a randomized clinical trial. Am J Orthod Dentofacial Orthop 2009;136(5):657–61.
22. Vanarsdall RL, Corn H. Soft-tissue management of labially positioned unerupted teeth. Am J Orthod 1977;72(1):53–64.
23. Kokich VG, Mathews DP. Surgical and orthodontic management of impacted teeth [review]. Dent Clin North Am 1993;37(2):181–204.
24. Crescini A, Clauser C, Giorgetti R, et al. Tunnel traction of infraosseous impacted maxillary canines. A three-year periodontal follow-up. Am J Orthod Dentofacial Orthop 1994;105(1):61–72.
25. Vermette ME, Kokich VG, Kennedy DB. Uncovering labially impacted teeth: apically positioned flap and closed-eruption techniques. Angle Orthod 1995;65(1):23–32 [discussion: 33].
26. Doufexi A, Mina M, Ioannidou E. Gingival overgrowth in children: epidemiology, pathogenesis, and complications. A literature review. J Periodontol 2005;76(1):3–10.
27. Parkin N, Benson PE, Thind B. Open versus closed surgical exposure of canine teeth that are displaced in the roof of the mouth. Cochrane Database Syst Rev 2008;(4):CD006966.
28. Zuccati G, Ghobadlu J, Nieri M, et al. Factors associated with the duration of forced eruption of impacted maxillary canines: a retrospective study. Am J Orthod Dentofacial Orthop 2006;130(3):349–56.

29. Iramaneerat S. The effect of two alternative methods of canine exposure upon subsequent duration of orthodontic treatment. Int J Paediatr Dent 1998;8(2):123–9.

30. Caminiti MF, Sandor GK, Giambattistini C, et al. Outcomes of the surgical exposure, bonding and eruption of 82 impacted maxillary canines. J Can Dent Assoc 1998;64(8):572–4, 576–9.

31. Becker A, Chaushu G, Chaushu S, et al. Analysis of failure in the treatment of impacted maxillary canines. Am J Orthod Dentofacial Orthop 2010;137(6):743–54.

32. Jacobs S. Localization of the unerupted maxillary canine: how to and when to. Am J Orthod Dentofacial Orthop 1999;115(3):314–22.

33. Sajnani AK, King NM. Retrospective audit of management techniques for treating impacted maxillary canines in children and adolescents over 27 year period. J Oral Maxillofac Surg 2011; 69(10):2494–9.

34. Neukam FW, Schultze-Mosgau S, Schliephake H, et al. Clinical and roentgenologic evaluation of the outcome of therapeutic tooth movement for occlusal adjustment. Fortschr Kiefer Gesichtschir 1995;40:97–9.

35. Fischer TJ. Orthodontic treatment acceleration with corticotomy-assisted exposure of palatally impacted canines. Angle Orthod 2007;77(3):417–20.

Office-Based Procedures for Unusual Impactions

Joshua Wolf, DDS*, Harry Dym, DDS

KEYWORDS

- Tooth impaction • Extraction • Coronectomy • Supernumerary teeth

KEY POINTS

- The order of frequency of tooth impaction includes mandibular and maxillary third molars, maxillary canines, mandibular premolars, mandibular canines, maxillary premolars, maxillary central incisors, maxillary lateral incisors, and mandibular second molars.
- Treatment of supernumerary teeth or impacted teeth should be based on clinical symptoms, location of the teeth, and a comprehensive examination of the impact of these teeth on neighboring teeth.
- In most cases, a diagnosis of supernumerary or impacted teeth is based on clinical symptoms and radiographic examination; the most common diagnoses are made by panoramic, occlusal, and periapical radiographs.
- Most unusual impacted teeth may be reached by the direct surgical approaches used to remove the commonly impacted sites, often requiring extensions of flaps and the removal of more bone.

Ectopic dentition refers to a tooth or teeth located away from the normal position within the jaws or in the vicinity of odontogenic structures. In contrast, heterotopic dentition includes a tooth or teeth present distantly into a site of an organ or tissue it does not normally occupy, such as in the case of the ovaries, mediastinum, and so forth. Unusual impacted teeth may include a supernumerary tooth, a tooth that migrated, or one that failed to erupt. The incidence of supernumerary teeth generally affects 0.1% to 1% of the population.[1]

Frequency and incidence of impacted teeth

The order of frequency of tooth impaction is mandibular and maxillary third molars, maxillary canines, mandibular premolars, mandibular canines, maxillary premolars, maxillary central incisors, maxillary lateral incisors, and mandibular second molars. Mandibular and maxillary first molars as well as maxillary second molars are very rarely impacted.

Etiology of supernumerary teeth

The cause of supernumerary teeth is not completely understood. One theory suggests that the supernumerary tooth is created either from a thin tooth bud that arises from the dental lamina near the permanent tooth bud or from splitting of the permanent bud itself. Heredity may also play a role in the occurrence of this anomaly, because supernumeraries are more common in the relatives of affected children than in the general population. However, the anomaly does not follow a simple Mendelian pattern. Although the cause of ectopic growth is not well understood, it has been attributed to obstruction at tooth eruption secondary to crowded dentition, persistent deciduous teeth, or exceptionally dense bone. Multiple supernumerary teeth are often associated with cleidocranial dysostosis but rare in those with no other associated diseases or syndromes.

It is theoretically possible for any tooth to follow an abortive eruptive path and become impacted within the dentoalveolar process or in remote or heterotopic anatomic sites, such as the nasal or sinus cavities, the mandibular ramus, or the inferior border of the mandible. In addition, teeth may not erupt into the dental arch owing to direct or indirect effects of cysts and neoplasm or to abnormal hereditary patterns of phenotypic expression. Therefore, it is prudent to perform a thorough clinical examination and obtain adequate radiographs when teeth do not appear according to the usual eruption schedule.

In most cases, a diagnosis of supernumerary or impacted teeth is based on clinical symptoms and radiographic examination. The most common diagnoses are made by panoramic, occlusal, and periapical radiographs.

However, radiographic film has the following 2 inevitable disadvantages:

1. Image overlap, which cannot reflect a 3-dimensional structure of the diseased region owing to a low-resolution ratio, and
2. Different degrees of distortion or amplification. In contrast, 3-dimensional computed tomographic (CT) imaging can reflect supernumerary teeth's shape, size, number, location, eruptive direction, and relative tissue conditions. Although there is still much debate as to when to order CT imaging from a medicolegal perspective, a CT's or Cone-Beam Computed

Disclosures: The author has nothing to disclose.

Department of Dentistry and Oral and Maxillofacial Surgery, The Brooklyn Hospital Center, 121 Dekalb Avenue, Box 187, Brooklyn, NY 11201, USA

* Corresponding author.

E-mail address: wolfjoshuac@gmail.com

http://dx.doi.org/10.1016/j.cxom.2013.06.001

Tomography's (CBCT) multidirectional and 3-dimensional display provides much information for treatment and surgical planning. One can assess the anatomic relationship between proximity of the inferior alveolar nerve (IAN) canal and the M3 roots and ascertain the location of the IAN canal relative to the roots.[2]

Treatment of supernumerary teeth or impacted teeth should be based on clinical symptoms, location of the teeth, and a comprehensive examination of the impact of these teeth on neighboring teeth. Supernumerary teeth need to be extracted in cases of clinical pathologic changes, orthodontic treatment, or where the tooth will be replaced with implants. As in cases of supernumerary teeth that are not in the dental arch, those with no clinical symptoms, or those that involve vital anatomic structures, such as intracranial, extraction of the teeth is not necessary, but further observation and follow-up are expected.

Most unusual impacted teeth may be reached by the direct surgical approaches used to remove the commonly impacted sites, often requiring extensions of flaps and the removal of more bone. This article discusses indirect and alternative techniques that the practitioner could use when the direct techniques would increase the chance of morbidity to the patient.

Mandibular locations

The issue of IAN involvement during the removal of the lower third molars is a clinical and medicolegal problem. Any technique that can reduce the possibility of this involvement is worthy of exploration. Coronectomy was developed as a relatively new preventive method to decrease the prevalence of IAN injury compared with the conventional total removal of the lower third molar.[3] A randomized controlled clinical trial published in 2009 has shown that coronectomy can significantly decrease the risk of an IAN deficit in high-risk cases.[4] The procedure has also been shown to be safe in terms of pain, infection rate, and dry socket, at least for the short term.[5]

The intention of coronectomy or deliberate root retention is that the part of the root intimately related to the IAN is undisturbed. However, enough of the root must be removed below the crest of the lingual and buccal plates of bone to enable bone to form over the retained roots as part of the normal healing process. It was also thought to be important not to mobilize the roots because they might damage the nerve. For this reason, complete transection of the crown and roots of the tooth was thought to be necessary.

The technique described by Pogrel and colleagues is as follows and is demonstrated in Fig. 1:

1. Following exposure of the crown, using a 701-type fissure bur, the crown of the tooth was transected at an angle of approximately 45°. The crown was totally transected so that it could be removed with tissue forceps alone and did not need to be fractured off the roots. This removal minimizes the possibility of mobilizing the roots. After removal of the crown of the tooth, the fissure bur is used to reduce the remaining root fragments so that the remaining roots are at least 3 mm below the crest of the lingual and buccal plates in all places, as can be seen in Fig. 2. An alternative technique is to use a round bur from a superior aspect and remove the crown and superior part of the roots by drilling

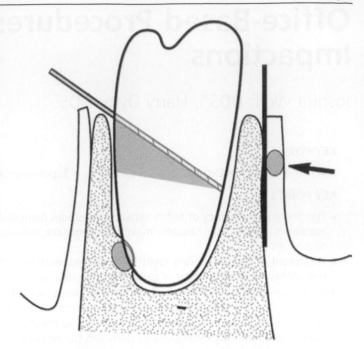

Fig. 1 Diagram showing the technique for removal of the lower right third molar. Note the angle of the bur at approximately 45° and lingual retractor protecting the lingual nerve (*arrow*). Shaded area of root on buccal side to be removed secondarily. (*From* Pogrel MA, Lee JS, Muff DF. Coronectomy: a technique to protect the inferior alveolar nerve. J Oral Maxillofac Surg 2004;62:1448; with permission.)

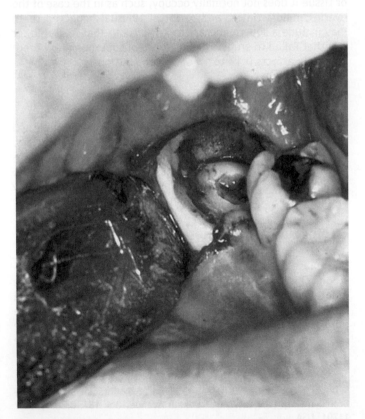

Fig. 2 Completeted coronectomy on lower right third molar. Note retained roots are 3 mm below the crest of bone and exposed pulp is untreated. (*From* Pogrel MA, Lee JS, Muff DF. Coronectomy: a technique to protect the inferior alveolar nerve. J Oral Maxillofac Surg 2004;62:1449; with permission.)

it away. In this case, only minimal lingual retraction may be required.

2. There is no attempt at root canal treatment or any other therapy to the exposed vital pulp of the tooth.
3. After a periosteal release, a watertight primary closure of the socket is performed with 1 or more vertical mattress sutures.

The following conditions should be considered when evaluating whether to perform a coronectomy:

1. Teeth with active infection around them, particularly infection involving the root portion, should be excluded from this technique.
2. Teeth that are mobile should be excluded from this technique because it is thought that the roots may act as a mobile foreign body and become a nidus for infection or migration.
3. Teeth that are horizontally impacted along the course of the IAN may be unsuitable for this technique because sectioning of the tooth itself could endanger the nerve. The technique is therefore better used for vertical, mesioangular, or distoangular impactions where the sectioning itself does not endanger the nerve.

Several studies comparing coronectomy with the total removal of the lower third molars have shown that an IAN deficit after coronectomy can be significantly decreased in high-risk cases. Root migration is a common finding in almost all studies on coronectomy of the lower third molars. As the root moves closer to the surface, it will be farther away from the nerve and carry a much smaller risk of nerve injury compared with removing the roots from their original situation. Sencimen and colleagues[6] reported a higher failure rate when they performed root canal treatment after coronectomy,

supporting the notion that the retained roots do not require any elective endodontics. Fig. 3 shows clinical examples of coronectomy with endodontic treatment and without endodontic treatment and the pulp left in place.

Marsupialization

Marsupialization may be advisable to allow eruption of an impacted or unerupted tooth associated with a cyst, if sufficient space exists. Two principal methods of treating a dentigerous cyst are removal and marsupialization. Excision is indicated when there is no likelihood of damaging anatomic structures, such as apices of vital teeth, maxillary sinus, or the IAN. Marsupialization can maintain the impacted tooth in its cavity and promote its eruption. Marsupialization is especially useful for dentigerous cysts with teeth displacement. The decompression can be performed by creating and protecting a surgical opening that unites the oral mucosa with the lining of the cyst. A biopsy is required to establish a reliable diagnosis of the lesion. Decompression of the cyst without tumor characteristics permits the displaced bone to regenerate and tooth to spontaneously erupt. New bone formation is stimulated because marsupialization decreases intracystic pressure. The major disadvantage of marsupialization is that pathologic tissue is left in situ, without a thorough histologic examination. In Fig. 4, Ertas and Yavuz[7] have shown a patient with a large cyst with displacement of 4 permanent teeth that was treated with marsupialization alone that resulted in eruption of all 4 displaced teeth. There is a close correlation between eruption and when the development of teeth roots had not been completed.[8]

In a marsupialization procedure, the cyst membrane is sutured to oral mucosa to create a window. A gauze iodoform pack can be inserted into the cyst cavity to keep it open. The packing is replaced biweekly and can be irrigated by the patient. The goal is for the tooth to erupt into the dental arch or

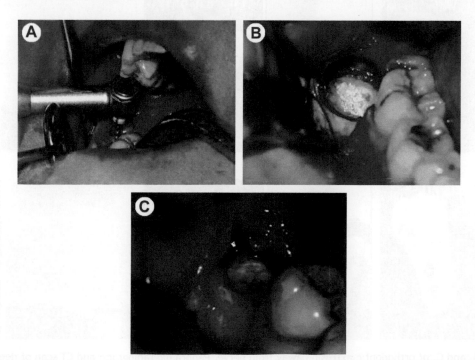

Fig. 3 (A) Removal of pulp and biomechanical preparation of roots. (B) Filling of canals with mineral trioxide aggregate. (C) Pulp was left in place in the control group. (*From* Sencimen M, Ortakoglu K, Aydin C, et al. Endodontic treatment during coronectomy. J Oral Maxillofac Surg 2010;68:2388; with permission.)

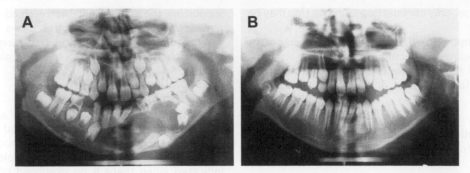

Fig. 4 (*A*) Panoramic radiograph showing the large dentigerous cyst and displaced teeth. (*B*) Thirty months after marsupialization, there has been no recurrence of the dentigerous cyst. (*From* Ertas U, Yavuz MS. Interesting eruption of 4 teeth associated with a large dentigerous cyst in mandible by only marsupialization. J Oral Maxillofac Surg 2003;61:728–30; with permission.)

into a position where damage to any anatomic structures is less likely.

Orthodontics

An orthodontic-surgical procedure can be useful for safe extraction of impacted third molars in the presence of high risks due to the tooth's close proximity to the mandibular canal. Different anchorage designs, wires, and bands have been developed to extrude impacted teeth as has been demonstrated by Bonetti and colleagues.[9] Fig. 5 demonstrates the clinical and radiographic benefits of the extrusion away from the canal. One of the disadvantages of this technique is that 2 surgeries are necessary: one to expose the

crown and place a bracket on one of the crown's surfaces, and second to remove the tooth after eruption from a safer position.

After the time needed for initial recovery of the soft tissues (about 1 week after the surgery), a rectangular stainless steel sectional wire is placed to activate the cantilever and allow the tooth to extrude, thus setting it apart from the mandibular canal. The cantilever must be untied, reshaped, and reactivated every 4 to 6 weeks. Once it has been verified that the roots are set apart from the canal, a second surgery, extraction of the tooth, can proceed. This operation should be quicker and easier than performing the extraction with the orthodontic extrusion and should carry less risk of complications, especially neurologic ones.

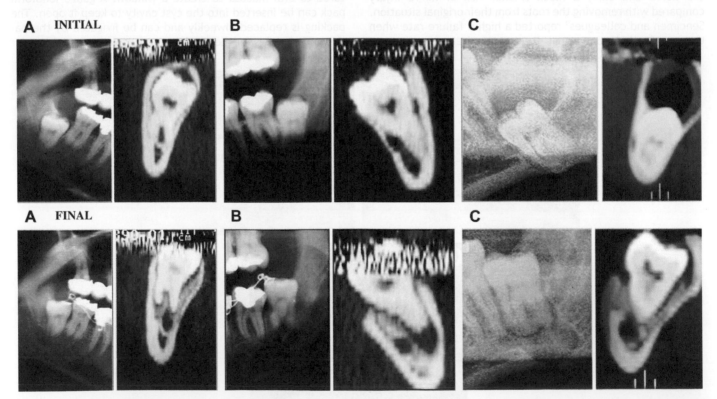

Fig. 5 3 cases, A, B, and C, of orthodontic extrusion away from nerve. Panoramic radiograph and CT scan of deep vertically impacted third molars before and after orthodontic extrusion. Notice the vertical movement of the impacted molars. (*From* Bonetti GA, Bendandi M, Checchi V, et al. Orthodontic extraction: riskless extraction of impacted lower third molars close to the mandibular canal. J Oral Maxillofac Surg 2007;65:2583; with permission.)

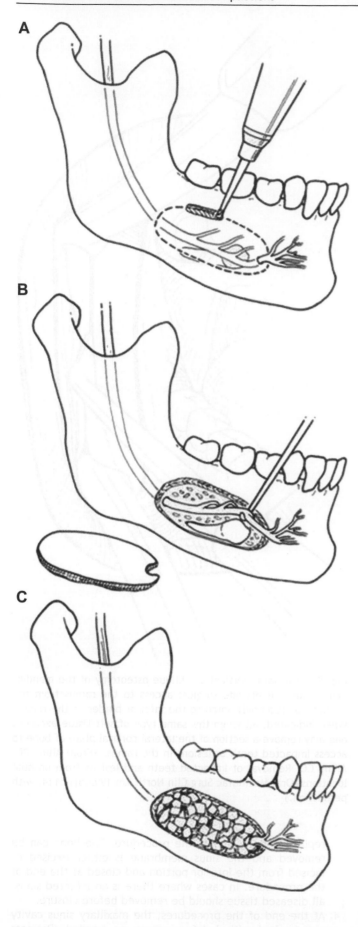

Removal of the mandible lateral bone

There will be indications to remove a cortical plate of bone from the lateral mandible to provide access below and above the inferior alveolar canal, as seen in Fig. 6.[10] The operation is performed as a transoral approach at the junction of the dentoalveolar mucoperiosteum and mucosa of the vestibule. A subperiosteal elevation is performed to expose the entire lateral cortex of the mandible. An osteotomy through the cortical bone is made with a piezoelectric or tapered bur. The plate is elevated with the assistance of a unibevel chisel and is preserved in normal saline. Access is provided to the cancellous area of the central portion of the body of the mandible. The thin cortical bone comprising the inferior alveolar canal may be removed if necessary with curettes and the neurovascular structures gently retracted away from the area of operation. Following the extraction of an impacted tooth, the IAN is replaced and the cortical bone is replaced using fixation plates and screw or the cortical bone can be cut up into small pieces and put into the defect.

Sagittal split osteotomy and vertical ramus osteotomy [vii] (slide 10, 11, 12, 13)

The surgical approach to an impacted tooth that has been displaced such a long distance and is located under the inferior alveolar can be removed by sagittal osteotomy of the mandibular ramus, as shown in Fig. 7. Advances in orthognathic surgery have allowed the use of these techniques in facial trauma, oncology, reconstructive surgery, and for the extraction of impacted teeth in unusual positions. An impacted tooth in the angle of the mandible and below the IAN can be extracted safely after a sagittal osteotomy of the mandibular ramus. Excellent surgical access is obtained, and postoperative complication rates and morbidity are low. It is not necessary to maintain the maxillomandibular fixation if the technique is performed unilaterally, and osteosynthesis techniques can be used, especially in a case where the skeletal relations of the bones have not been modified. The vertical ramus osteotomy can be used for removal of teeth in the posterior ramus from the sigmoid notch to the inferior border, as seen in Fig. 8.

Maxillary locations

In the maxilla, lesions may be located in the intrasinal, intranasal, and introrbital positions. Surgical approaches to these areas may be by routes other than through the dentoalveolar process.

Fig. 6 Removal of lateral cortical bone of the mandible will give surgical access to the body of the mandible. (*A*) The osteotomy of the lateral cortical plate may be performed with a bur. (*B*) The inferior alveolar neurovascular structures are lifted off the impacted supernumerary tooth. (*C*) Following removal of the tooth, the cortical plate, which had been preserved in normal saline, is fragmented and replaced. Note: This operation may not be indicated if there is inadequate cross-sectional substance to the mandible to provide structural integrity during the 2- to 3-month normal postoperative repairing phases. (*From* Alling RD, Alling CC. Removal of impacted teeth and lesions from unusual locations. Oral Maxillofac Surg Clin North Am 1995;5(1):113; with permission.)

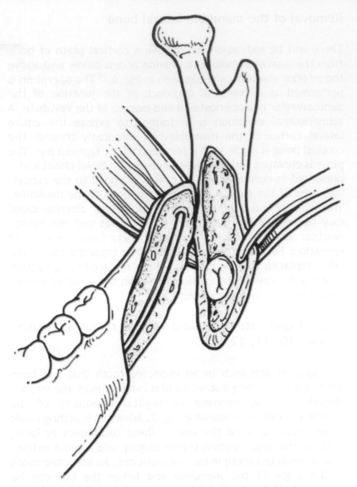

Fig. 7 Sagittal split osteotomy of the mandibular ramus provides surgical access to the posterior body and to the lower half of the ramus of the mandible. (*From* Alling RD, Alling CC. Removal of impacted teeth and lesions from unusual locations. Oral Maxillofac Surg Clin North Am 1995;5(1):114; with permission.)

Caldwell-Luc transoral sinus surgery

The Caldwell-Luc operation has a long history in the treatment of sinus disease. It was first described by George Caldwell in 1893 and Henri Luc in 1897 as a surgical approach to maxillary sinus disease. This procedure was a mainstay of treatment of chronic and recurrent maxillary sinusitis until the introduction of functional endoscopic sinus surgery for improving physiologic drainage at the natural ostia. Impacted or displaced teeth or other pathologic entities can be removed using this procedure, as seen in Fig. 9. The standard procedure shown in Fig. 10 involves the following steps[11]:

1. Gingivobuccal fold incision or intrasulcular incision with vertical releasing cuts.
2. If the patient had an oroantral communication, the incision was designed to create a buccal advanced flap to cover the defect. The infraorbital nerve is carefully protected during periosteal elevation. A bone window is made at the canine fossa or over the lesion or impacted tooth, which is determined before the surgery.
3. Opening the bone of the sinus can be performed with instruments based on surgeon preference. To enter the sinus cavity, a bone sinus composite flap can be used that can be

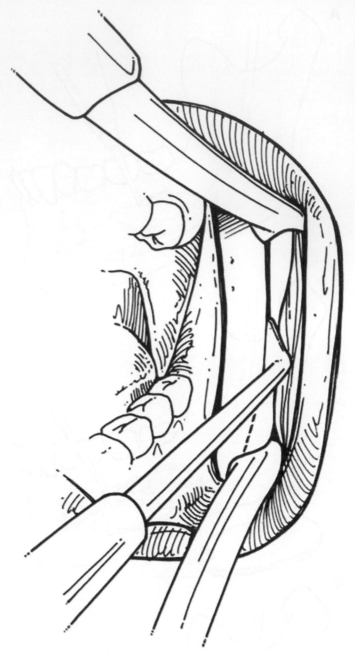

Fig. 8 Transoral vertical or oblique osteotomy of the mandibular ramus will provide surgical access to the ramus from the mandibular (sigmoid) notch to the inferior border of the ramus. When indicated, although this same type of soft tissue excision, one may remove a section of the lateral cortical plate of bone to access impacted teeth or lesions in the ramus. (*From* Alling RD, Alling CC. Removal of impacted teeth and lesions from unusual locations. Oral Maxillofac Surg Clin North Am 1995;5(1):114; with permission.)

replaced at the end of the procedure. The bone can be removed and the sinus membrane is either excised or incised from the inferior portion and closed at the end of the procedure. In cases where there is an infected sinus, all diseased tissue should be removed before closure.

4. At the end of the procedures, the maxillary sinus cavity was packed with iodoform gauze as needed. Patients should be instructed to use sinus precaution for 2 weeks.

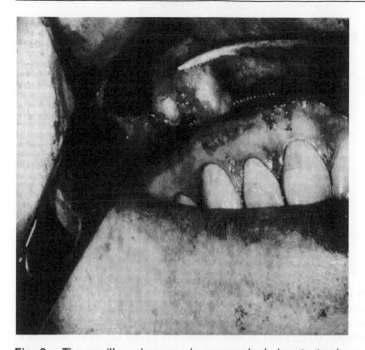

Fig. 9 The maxillary sinus may be approached via ostectomies through the anterior surface of the maxilla for removal of teeth located in or displaced into the sinus. (*From* Alling RD, Alling CC. Removal of impacted teeth and lesions from unusual locations. Oral Maxillofac Surg Clin North Am 1995;5(1):117; with permission.)

Patients with sinus packing should return for removal of the iodoform gauze packing on the fifth day after surgery.

The Caldwell-Luc antrostomy approach also tends to leave bony defects in the anterior and lateral walls of the maxillary sinus when large tumors are removed.

These osseous defects might not regenerate, leaving permanent voids in the bones of these areas. If these voids are large enough, they can allow collapse of the overlying soft tissues in the space normally occupied by the walls of the maxillary sinus.

Midfacial downfracture procedures

Le ForteI down-fracture of the maxilla can give generous access to the maxillary sinus and nasal areas.[12] For surgeons who routinely perform this operation for various dentofacial deformities, it is a relatively easy way to gain the needed access for tooth removal. This procedure also provides exposure to manage tooth removal and hemorrhage control properly in the lateral nasal, posterior maxillary, and orbital floor regions. The Le Fort I down-fracture approach can avoid some of these problems. The Le Fort I down-fracture provides excellent exposure of a tumor or tooth and avoids sacrificing large amounts of bone as seen in the removal of a large odontoma in Fig. 11. The postoperative healing is predictable, without oroantral fistula formation.

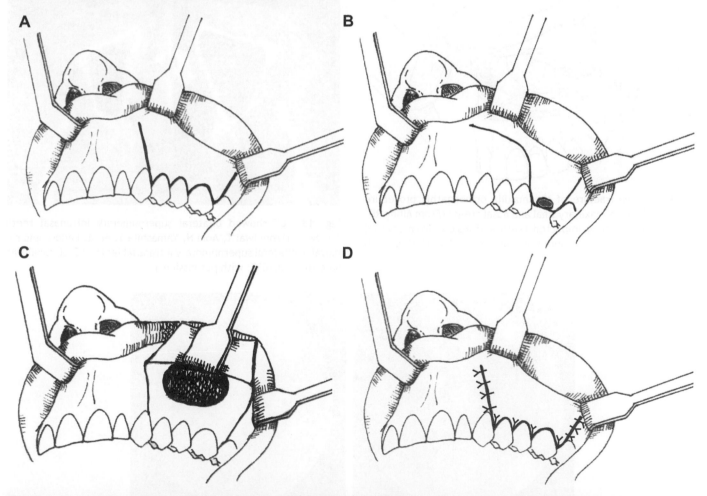

Fig. 10 (*A*) An intrasulcular incision with 2 vertical releasing cuts was made at the cyst/tumor-involving area. (*B*) A buccal advanced flap to repair the oroantral communication was designed. (*C*) A bone window was made at the canine fossa. No inferior meatal antrostomy was made at the end of the operation. (*D*) The intraoral incision was closed with absorbable suture. (*From* Huang YC, Chen WH. Caldwell-Luc operation without inferior meatal antrostomy: a retrospective study of 50 cases. J Oral Maxillofac Surg 2012;70:2081; with permission.)

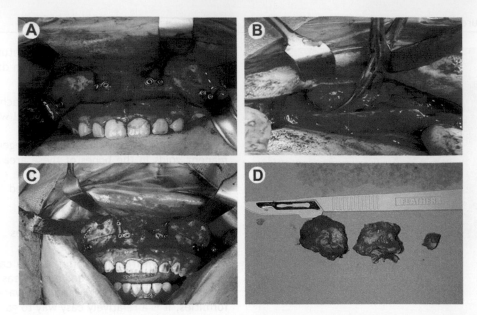

Fig. 11 (*A*) Titanium mini-plates positioned and Le Fort osteotomy level drawn on anterior and lateral surfaces of maxilla. (*B*) Maxilla down-fractured at Le Fort I level, and odontoma visualized in right posterior aspect of maxillary sinus. This approach allows the surgeon the opportunity to reach into the maxillary sinus and more easily remove the mass. (*C*) Preadapted titanium mini-plates have re-established preoperative occlusion postoperatively. (*D*) Enucleated complex odontoma. (*From* Korpi JT, Kainulainen VT, Sándor GK, et al. Removal of large complex odontoma using Le Fort I osteotomy. J Oral Maxillofac Surg 2009;67:2020; with permission.)

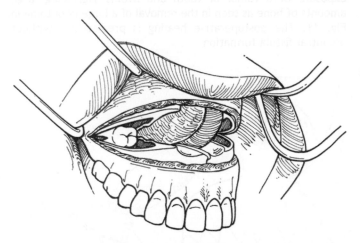

Fig. 12 Down-fracture of the maxilla orthognathic procedure gives access to the maxillary sinal and nasal areas. (*From* Alling RD, Alling CC. Removal of impacted teeth and lesions from unusual locations. Oral Maxillofac Surg Clin North Am 1995;5(1):116; with permission.)

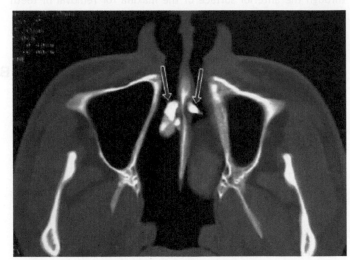

Fig. 13 CT showed bilateral supernumerary intranasal teeth (*arrows*). (*From* Iwai T, Aoki N, Yamashita Y, et al. Endoscopic removal of bilateral supernumerary intranasal teeth. J Oral Maxillofac Surg 2012;70;1032; with permission.)

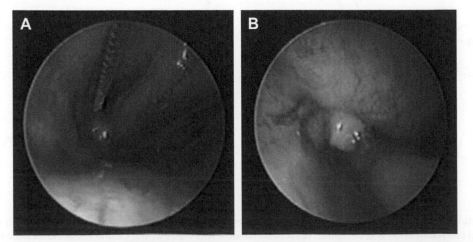

Fig. 14 (*A*) Endoscopic removal of left supernumerary intranasal tooth. (*B*) Endoscopic view of left supernumerary intranasal teeth. (*From* Iwai T, Aoki N, Yamashita Y, et al. Endoscopic removal of bilateral supernumerary intranasal teeth. J Oral Maxillofac Surg 2012:70;1033; with permission.)

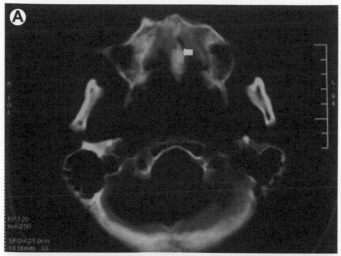

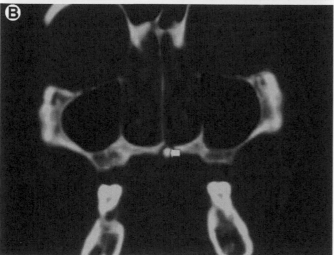

Fig. 15 CT images of a supernumerary tooth (*arrows*) in the palatine bone in the (*A*) axial and (*B*) coronal planes. (*From* Xu GZ, Yang C, Chuang QY, et al. Embedded supernumerary teeth in the horizontal plate of palatine bone: report of 2 rare cases. J Oral Maxillofac Surg 2011;69:1296; with permission.)

The Le Fort I down-fracture approach provides superior visualization compared with the Caldwell-Luc antrostomy approach, particularly for tumors in the posterior maxilla, which can be difficult to see.

To use this procedure to remove lesions or teeth, a routine Le Fort I osteotomy incision is made to expose the maxilla. An osteotomy is made from the right to the left pterygoid plates with an oscillating saw and chisel technique, and the maxilla is down-fractured with finger pressure in a routine fashion. The maxilla in its down-fractured position can be seen in Fig. 12, giving excellent access to the nasal and sinus areas. The maxilla is repositioned in its previous position and secured with mini-plates.

Rare impaction sites

Intranasal teeth
The diagnosis of an intranasal tooth can be confirmed clinically and radiologically. An intranasal tooth is often a hard white mass clinically and is sometimes covered completely by nasal mucosa and surrounded by granulation tissue and necrotic debris.

Radiography is useful for the diagnosis because intranasal teeth are identified as radiopaque lesions. Although panoramic radiographs can provide detailed information about the condition of dentition and whether the intranasal tooth is supernumerary, deciduous, or a permanent tooth, such radiographs are not always sufficient to identify intranasal teeth off the midline. Because conventional radiologic examination may not be able to confirm supernumerary intranasal teeth precisely, CT, as shown in Fig. 13, is useful to identify supernumerary intranasal teeth. Supernumerary intranasal teeth should be removed as soon as they are detected because of potential morbidity.[13] However, in children the most appropriate time for removal is when the roots of the permanent teeth have completely formed, to minimize the risk of developmental injury to the dentition. Although some intranasal teeth may be asymptomatic, such intranasal teeth should be removed or at least followed radiographically. Supernumerary intranasal teeth may be removed by a transnasal approach or intraoral approach according to site of the intranasal teeth. The transnasal approach is often less invasive, but this approach under direct vision with a nasal speculum and head light cannot provide sufficient visualization to remove supernumerary intranasal teeth in the posterior region of the nasal cavity. To overcome the problem, endoscopy has recently been used to remove intranasal teeth as a minimally invasive surgery. Endoscopic removal of intranasal teeth can provide good illumination, better visualization,

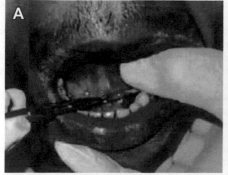

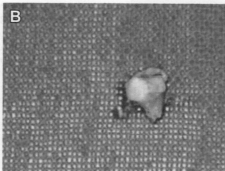

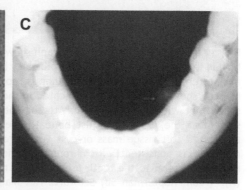

Fig. 16 (*A*) Preoperative intraoral view. (*B*) Excised mass. (*C*) Occlusal radiograph showing radiopacity on left side. (*From* Gupta DS, Tandon PN, Sharma S, et al. Intraglandular tooth—rare case report of tooth in submandibular salivary gland duct. J Oral Maxillofac Surg 2011;69:e305—6; with permission.)

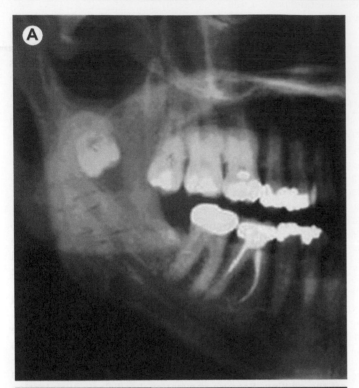

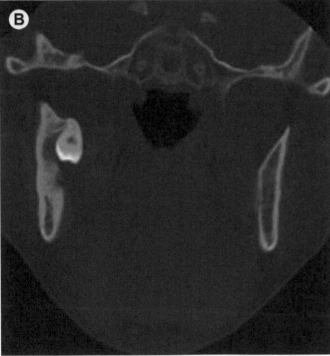

Fig. 17 (*A*) The panoramic radiograph shows an inverted molar, high in the mandibular ramus. A radiolucency below the crown was misinterpreted by a previous examiner as representing a cyst. (*B*) CT scan shows that the tooth is located in the pterygomandibular space, not within the mandible. Attachment to the mandible is seen near the root apex, just beneath the sigmoid notch. No associated soft tissue mass or cyst is apparent. Sclerosis of the mandible is consistent with chronic infection. Thinning of the mandible lateral to the tooth produced the radiolucency seen in (*A*). (*From* Kupferman SB, Schwartz HC. Malposed teeth in the pterygomandibular space: report of 2 cases. J Oral Maxillofac Surg 2008;66:168; with permission.)

and precise dissection with preservation of surrounding tissue compared with a conventional approach, as demonstrated in Fig. 14.[14]

Fig. 15 shows teeth as seen in the horizontal palate,[15] Fig. 16 depicts the submandibular salivary duct,[16] and Fig. 17 displays the pterygomandibular space.[17]

Cases in the literature have reported teeth that were in locations associated with the oral cavity, but do not seem to have been displaced by a cyst or a tumor. Although the approach to their removal of these teeth was a direct approach using incisions used for other oral surgery procedures, the oral surgeon should be aware that teeth can arise in unusual locations and the decision to remove them should be made on a case-by-case basis.

References

1. Thawley SE, LaFerriere KA. Supernumerary nasal tooth. Laryngoscope 1977;87:1770.
2. Susarla MS. Dodson: preoperative computed tomography imaging in the management of impacted mandibular third molars. J Oral Maxillofac Surg 2007;65:83–8.
3. Pogrel MA, Lee JS, Muff DF. Coronectomy: a technique to protect the inferior alveolar nerve. J Oral Maxillofac Surg 2004;62:1447.
4. Leung YY, Cheung LK. Safety of coronectomy versus excision of wisdom teeth: a randomized controlled trial. Oral Surg Oral Med Oral Pathol Oral Radiol Endod 2009;108:821.
5. Leung YY, Cheung LK. Coronectomy of the lower third molar is safe within the first 3 years. J Oral Maxillofac Surg 2012;70:1515–22.
6. Sencimen M, Ortakoglu K, Aydin C, et al. Is endodontic treatment necessary during coronectomy procedure? J Oral Maxillofac Surg 2010;68:2385.
7. Ertas U, Yavuz MS. Interesting eruption of 4 teeth associated with a large dentigerous cyst in mandible by only marsupialization. J Oral Maxillofac Surg 2003;61:728–30.
8. Miyawaki S, Hyomoto M, Tsubauchi J, et al. Eruption speed and rate of angulation change of a cyst-associated mandibular second premolar after marsupialization of a dentigerous cyst. Am J Orthod Dentofacial Orthop 1999;116:578.
9. Bonetti GA, Bendandi M, Checchi V. Orthodontic extraction: riskless extraction of impacted lower third molars close to the mandibular canal. J Oral Maxillofac Surg 2007;65:2580–6.
10. Alling RD, Alling III CC. Removal of impacted teeth and lesions from unusual locations. Oral Maxillofac Surg Clin North Am 1993;5:111–9.
11. Huang YC, Chen WH. Caldwell-luc operation without inferior meatal antrostomy: a retrospective study of 50 cases. J Oral Maxillofac Surg 2012;70:2080–4.
12. Korpi JT, Kainulainen VT, Sandor GK, et al. Removal of large complex odontoma using Le Fort I osteotomy. J Oral Maxillofac Surg 2009;67:2018–21.
13. Lee JH. A nasal tooth associated with septal perforation: a rare occurrence. Eur Arch Otorhinolaryngol 2006;263:1055.
14. Iwai T, Aoki N, Yamashita Y, et al. Endoscopic removal of bilateral supernumerary intranasal teeth. J Oral Maxillofac Surg 2012;70:1030–4.
15. Xu GZ, Yang C, Chuang QY, et al. Embedded supernumerary teeth in the horizontal plate of palatine bone: report of 2 rare cases. J Oral Maxillofac Surg 2011;69(5):1295–300.
16. Gupta DS, Tandon PN, Sharma S, et al. Intraglandular tooth—rare case report of tooth in submandibular salivary gland duct. J Oral Maxillofac Surg 2011;69:e305–7.
17. Kupferman SB, Schwartz HC. Malposed teeth in the pterygomandibular space: report of 2 cases. J Oral Maxillofac Surg 2008;66:167–9.

Coronectomy

Indications, Outcomes, and Description of Technique

Jacob Gady, DMD, MD [a], Mark C. Fletcher, DMD, MD [a,b],*

KEYWORDS

- Coronectomy • Third molars • Inferior alveolar nerve

KEY POINTS

- Coronectomy is considered a reasonable and safe treatment alternative for patients who demonstrate elevated risk for injury to the inferior alveolar nerve with the removal of third molars.
- The procedure has been documented in the oral and maxillofacial surgery literature as a treatment alternative to extraction of third molar in patients considered at elevated risk for permanent nerve injury.
- Coronectomy is particularly appropriate for patients who are older than 25 years and who report low tolerance for the possibility of posttreatment neurosensory deficit at the consultation.
- Appropriate patient selection for coronectomy is paramount.
- Periodic follow-up assessments are required, and patient compliance is essential.

Coronectomy was first described by Ecuyer and Debien in 1984 as an alternative procedure to traditional extraction of third molars.[1] Several reports have been published since regarding the technique, indications, efficacy, and outcome of this procedure. Most recently, it has been investigated as an alternative to traditional surgical extraction of third molars, particularly for those with an increased risk of damage to the inferior alveolar nerve (IAN). Several studies have demonstrated that coronectomy does significantly decrease the risk of iatrogenic injury to the IAN, with some studies also suggesting a lower complication rate. This article discusses the indications for coronectomy, the author's technique, and the complications and outcomes of this procedure.

Indications

The main indication for performing a coronectomy is to prevent iatrogenic injury to the IAN when removing a third molar. Therefore, the ability to determine whether the IAN is at high risk is paramount and should be well understood.

The frequency of IAN damage after extraction of a third molar ranges anywhere from 0.4% to 8.4%.[2-5] Panoramic radiographs are traditionally used in the preoperative evaluation of patients who will undergo surgical extraction of mandibular teeth. Increasingly, computed tomography scanning is used to evaluate the relationship of the tooth to the IAN in 3 dimensions, but is not yet the standard of care, owing to cost and the increased exposure of the patient to radiation. Certain radiographic features that depict an increased risk of iatrogenic IAN damage when extracting third molars include darkening of the root, narrowing of the apices, deflection of the root, diversion of the IAN canal, narrowing of the IAN canal, and interruption of the white line of the IAN canal.[2,6] Coronectomy may decrease the incidence of damage to the IAN in these cases of increased risk.

Pogrel and colleagues[7] performed 50 coronectomies on 41 patients who were at significantly increased risk of IAN damage from panoramic radiographic assessment, and found no postoperative cases of inferior alveolar nerve involvement. Similar results were reported by Leung and Cheung,[8] who performed 171 coronectomies and 178 surgical extractions (controls) of third molars on 231 patients. Nine patients in the control group presented with IAN sensory deficit versus 1 patient in the coronectomy group, demonstrating a statistically significant decrease in IAN damage using coronectomy for high-risk patients.[8]

Contraindications

The success of coronectomy depends on the survival of the retained root fragments with the successful formation of osteocementum and bone over the roots. Any tooth with active caries into the pulp, or demonstrating periapical abnormality should not be considered for coronectomy. Horizontally impacted teeth and teeth associated with tumors or large cysts should be excluded. The coronectomy procedure can otherwise be accomplished with vertically positioned, mesially tilted, and distally angulated teeth. Other local factors excluding coronectomy are patients scheduled for an osteotomy in the future. Patients excluded for systemic reasons from undergoing coronectomy include immunocompromised patients (chemotherapy, AIDS, radiation therapy, immunomodulating drug

Disclosures: The authors have nothing to disclose.

[a] Department of Craniofacial Sciences, Division of Oral and Maxillofacial Surgery, University of Connecticut School of Dental Medicine, 263 Farmington Avenue, Farmington, CT 06030, USA

[b] Avon Oral and Maxillofacial Surgery, 34 Dale Road, Suite 105, Avon, CT 06001-3659, USA

* Corresponding author. 34 Dale Road, Suite #105, Avon, CT 06001, USA.

E-mail address: markcfletcher@att.net

Atlas Oral Maxillofacial Surg Clin N Am 21 (2013) 221-226

1061-3315/13/$ - see front matter © 2013 Elsevier Inc. All rights reserved.

http://dx.doi.org/10.1016/j.cxom.2013.05.008

therapy, and so forth), poorly controlled diabetics, and those patients who are to undergo radiation therapy.[7–9]

Technique

The technique used by the authors and described here is similar to that described in the literature, for example by Pogrel and colleagues.[7]

1. First the patients are evaluated radiographically for root proximity to the IAN. If the patient is at significant increased risk for damage to the IAN, the option of coronectomy is discussed as an alternative to third-molar extraction. Criteria for selection involves the degree of root development, the degree of associated abnormality, the age of the patient, and patient tolerance for the potential of sustaining permanent neurosensory disturbance (Fig. 1A–D).
2. Once coronectomy has been decided upon for treatment, informed consent is obtained. Included in the consent process is a thorough discussion of the rationale for coronectomy. Risks including, but not limited to, infection, neurosensory disturbance, coronal migration of retained root fragments requiring surgical retrieval, and the potential need for additional surgical procedures are discussed. The possibility that extraction of the tooth may be necessary in the event of extensive decay, active infection, and mobility of retained roots is also included in the consent process.
3. IAN blocks including long buccal infiltration are accomplished with 2% lidocaine with 1:100,000 epinephrine and 0.5% bupivacaine with 1:100,000 epinephrine. A full-thickness mucoperiosteal incision is elevated with posterior buccal release. If necessary, a conservative buccal trough is made using a #6 round carbide bur on a nitrogen-driven surgical hand piece, allowing access to the cementoenamel junction of the tooth. Care is exercised to maintain as much crestal bone height as possible by minimizing the width of the buccal trough. After exposure is obtained, a 701 fissure bur is used and a horizontal/transverse cut is made through the tooth at the level of the cementoenamel junction. Visualization is important to ensure adequate sectioning of the crown without perforation through the lingual bone plate. The crown is delicately fractured and separated from the residual roots of the

tooth using a straight elevator. Effort is directed at minimizing any mobilization of the residual roots. On removal of the crown, any sharp fragments of retained tooth structure are smoothed down with a 2.3-mm diameter diamond round bur with simultaneous copious saline irrigation. The remaining enamel is typically reduced approximately 3 mm below the buccal crest of alveolar bone (Fig. 2A–J).

   a. Root canal treatment is not indicated during coronectomy. Sencimen and colleagues[10] found that patients having coronectomy with root canal treatment had a much higher infection rate than those patients who underwent coronectomy without root canal treatment. Seven of the 8 patients undergoing root canal treatment developed postoperative infections, whereas only 1 of 8 patients in the control group developed an infection. The investigators suggested that mobilization of the root during root canal therapy and/or prolonged procedure time may contribute to the higher infection rate in the study group.
4. After the coronectomy is completed, a dental curette is used for removal of any and all follicular soft tissue in the surgical bony defect. Any grossly visible exposed pulpal soft tissue is curetted. A bone file is used to smooth the bone edges along the socket defect and buccal bone trough. The incision is copiously irrigated with saline, and a small amount of doxycycline powder (doxycycline hyclate, 50 mg capsules; Watson Laboratories, Corona, CA) is applied topically to the surgical site before closure with chromic suture. Primary closure is desirable whenever possible, and may involve making a releasing incision distal to the second molar to facilitate closure. An immediate postoperative panoramic radiograph is obtained for a baseline assessment of the retained root fragment (Fig. 3A–F).
5. Postoperatively, patients are placed on a 1-week course of antibiotic therapy. Typically penicillin VK, 500 mg by mouth 4 times daily or clindamycin 300 mg by mouth 3 times daily (in penicillin allergic patients) is used. Chlorhexidine gluconate oral rinse 0.12% 3 times daily for 10 days is prescribed postoperatively. Analgesia is accomplished with hydrocodone/acetaminophen and nonsteroidal anti-inflammatories, as in patients who have had a third molar extracted. Patients are scheduled for a follow-up visit at approximately 10 days after surgery, and are given an

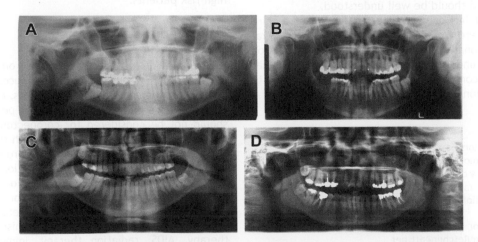

Fig. 1 Patients noted to be at elevated risk for injury to the inferior alveolar nerve. (*A*) A 41-year-old woman presenting with pericoronitis, teeth #17 and #32. (*B*) A 69-year-old woman presenting with pericoronitis and caries, tooth #17. (*C*) A 41-year-old man presenting with pericoronitis, tooth #17. (*D*) A 41-year-old woman presenting with pericoronitis and infection, tooth #32.

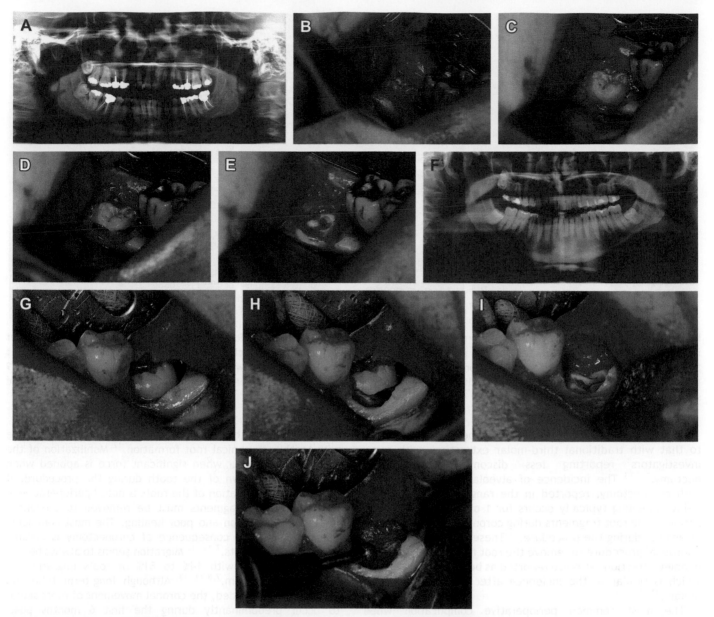

Fig. 2 Photographic documentation of the coronectomy procedure using the author's technique, involving 2 patients. Patient I.P. is a 41-year-old woman who presented with pericoronitis and infection associated with impacted tooth #32. Patient H.N. is a 41-year-old man who presented with pericoronitis associated with tooth #17. (*A*) Patient I.P.: pretreatment panoramic radiograph (also seen in Fig. 1D). (*B*) Patient I.P.: surgical exposure of tooth #32. (*C*) Patient I.P.: trough formation with #6 round bur. (*D*) Patient I.P.: horizontal cut made with 701 tapered fissure bur. (*E*) Patient I.P.: after removal of crown of tooth #32. (*F*) Patient H.N.: pretreatment panoramic radiograph (also seen in Fig. 1C). (*G*) Patient H.N.: trough formation around tooth #17 with #6 round bur. (*H*) Patient H.N.: horizontal cut made with 701 tapered fissure bur. (*I*) Patient H.N.: after removal of crown, tooth #17. (*J*) Patient H.N.: residual roots smoothed with a 2.3-mm diameter diamond round bur.

irrigation syringe for cleansing of the surgical site at that time. Patients are instructed to return for reevaluation at 6 months postoperatively. A periodontal assessment and panoramic radiograph is obtained at the 6-month post-treatment visit. In the author's practice, an immediate posttreatment panoramic radiograph is obtained for base-line assessment, and a subsequent panoramic radiograph or periapical radiograph is obtained at 6 months posttreat-ment to assess for coronal migration of roots, potential abscess formation, bone formation over the residual root fragments, and overall healing. It is the author's opinion that this radiographic protocol is warranted given the

reduced incidence of permanent neurosensory disturbance in these patients (Figs. 4–7).

Complications

Complications after coronectomy are similar to those of traditional third-molar surgery, which are well known to oral and maxillofacial surgeons: bleeding, infection, pain, IAN damage, alveolar osteitis, and poor healing. Complications unique to coronectomy include mobilization of the roots during the procedure and postoperative migration of the roots.

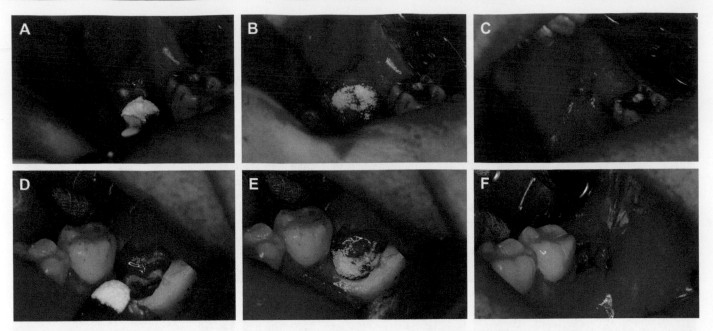

Fig. 3 Completion of coronectomy procedures using the authors' technique on patients I.P. and H.N. (*A*) Patient I.P.: doxycycline powder is applied topically to residual root with #9 periosteal elevator. (*B*) Patient I.P.: doxycycline powder in surgical site. (*C*) Patient I.P.: primary closure of surgical site with 3-0 chromic suture. (*D*) Patient H.N.: doxycycline powder applied topically to residual root with #9 periosteal elevator. (*E*) Patient H.N.: doxycycline powder in surgical site. (*F*) Patient H.N.: primary closure of surgical site with 3-0 chromic suture.

Postoperative discomfort does not appear to be different to that with traditional third-molar extraction, with some investigators reporting less discomfort with coronectomy.[11–13] The incidence of alveolar osteitis is similar with coronectomy, reported in the range of 10% to 12%.[13] Delayed healing typically occurs for 1 of 2 reasons: mobilization of the root fragments during coronectomy or retention of enamel during the procedure.[11] These patients require an additional procedure to remove the root fragment or retained enamel. Infection rates are reported as between 1% and 5.2%, which is similar to the incidence after extraction of third molars.[11–13]

The most common perioperative complication when performing coronectomy is mobilization of the root fragment.[7,11,12] Patients at higher risk are females and those with teeth with conical root formation.[12] Mobilization of the roots will also occur when significant force is applied when fracturing the crown of the tooth during the procedure. If inadvertent mobilization of the roots is noted perioperatively, the mobile root fragments must be removed to prevent a foreign-body reaction and poor healing. The most commonly reported long-term consequence of coronectomy is coronal migration of the roots.[7,11–13] Migration seems to always be in a coronal direction, with 14% to 81% of roots migrating on average 2 to 4 mm.[7,8,11–13] Although long-term follow-up studies are still needed, the coronal movement of roots seems to occur predominantly during the first 6 months postoperatively and slows down thereafter.

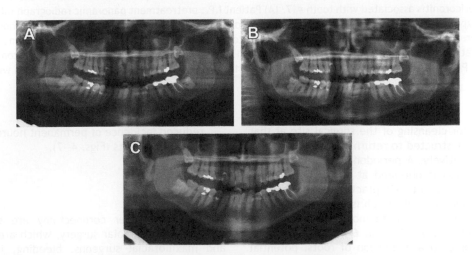

Fig. 4 Patient W.B. is a 62-year-old man with a history of pain, pericoronitis, and caries associated with tooth #17. He was planned for coronectomy on tooth #17. (*A*) Preoperative panoramic radiograph. (*B*) Immediate postoperative panoramic radiograph. (*C*) Panoramic radiograph obtained 8 months postoperatively.

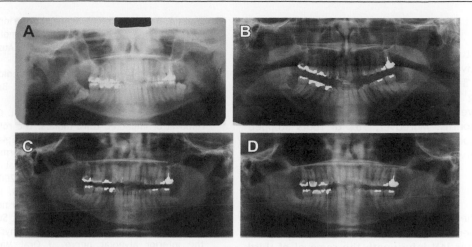

Fig. 5 Patient K.N. is a 41-year-old woman who presented with pericoronitis associated with teeth #17 and #32. She was planned for coronectomies on both teeth. (*A*) Preoperative panoramic radiograph (also seen in Fig. 1A). (*B*) Immediate postoperative panoramic radiograph. (*C*) Panoramic radiograph obtained 6 months postoperatively. (*D*) Panoramic radiograph obtained 27 months postoperatively. Note coronal migration of residual roots away from radiographic inferior alveolar nerve canals.

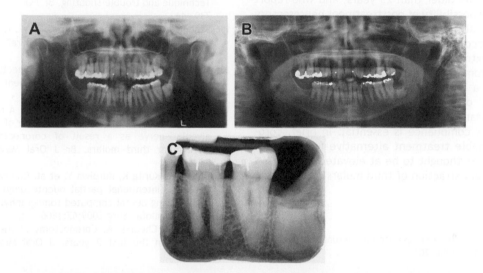

Fig. 6 Patient B.A. is a 69-year-old woman with caries and pericoronitis associated with tooth #17. She was planned for coronectomy. (*A*) Preoperative panoramic radiograph. (*B*) Immediate postoperative panoramic radiograph. (*C*) Periapical radiograph obtained from restorative dentist 7 months postoperatively. The patient refused to return for 6-month postoperative panoramic radiograph, stating "lack of symptoms."

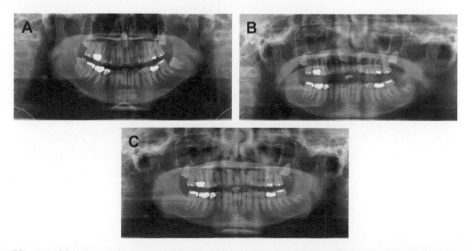

Fig. 7 Patient B.P. is a 58-year-old woman who presented with pericoronitis associated with tooth #17 and caries associated with tooth #32. She was planned for coronectomy on tooth #17 and extraction of tooth #32. (*A*) Preoperative panoramic radiograph. (*B*) Immediate postoperative panoramic radiograph. (*C*) Panoramic radiograph 6 months postoperatively. Note bone regeneration over the residual roots of tooth #17.

Outcomes

There are several studies reported in the literature with 12-month postoperative follow-up data. However, few long-term studies exist. A 3-year follow-up study published in 2012 by Leung and Cheung[14] found no increase in the incidence of infection, pain, development of abnormalities, and root eruption after 12 months. Moreover, 75% of roots stopped migrating 12 to 24 months postoperatively, and there was no migration of roots between 24 and 36 months.

Summary

It is the opinion of the authors that coronectomy is a reasonable and safe treatment alternative for patients who demonstrate elevated risk for IAN injury with the removal of third molars. The procedure has been documented in the oral and maxillofacial surgery literature as a treatment alternative to third-molar extraction in patients considered at elevated risk for permanent nerve injury. Coronectomy is particularly appropriate for patients older than 25 years, and who report low tolerance for the possibility of posttreatment neurosensory deficit at the consultation. The procedure is straightforward, and postoperative recovery is comparable with that of traditional third-molar extraction. Lastly, appropriate patient selection for coronectomy is paramount. Although not typical, patients must have a realistic understanding that additional surgery (eg, removal of residual roots or treatment of infection) may be necessary. Periodic follow-up assessments are required and patient compliance is essential. In brief, coronectomy is a reasonable treatment alternative for appropriately selected patients thought to be at elevated risk for IAN injury associated with extraction of third molars.

References

1. Ecuyer J, Debien J. Deductions operatoires. Actual Odontostomatol (Paris) 1984;38(148):695—701.

2. Smith A, Barry SE, Chiong AY, et al. Inferior alveolar nerve damage following removal of mandibular third molar teeth. a prospective study using panoramic radiography. Aust Dent J 1997;42(3): 149—52.

3. Rood JP, Shehab BA. The radiological prediction of inferior alveolar nerve injury during third molar surgery. Br J Oral Maxillofac Surg 1990;28:20—5.

4. Sisk AL, Hammer WB, Shelton DW, et al. Complications following removal of impacted third molars: the role of the experience of the surgeon. J Oral Maxillofac Surg 1986;44:855—9.

5. Gulicher D, Gerlach KL. Sensory impairment of the lingual and inferior alveolar nerves following removal of impacted mandibular third molars. Int J Oral Maxillofac Surg 2001;30:306—12.

6. Sedaghatfar M, August MA, Dodson TB. Panoramic radiographic findings as predictors of inferior alveolar nerve exposure following third molar extraction. J Oral Maxillofac Surg 2005;63:3—7.

7. Pogrel MA, Lee JS, Muff DF. Coronectomy: a technique to protect the inferior alveolar nerve. J Oral Maxillofac Surg 2004;62: 1447—52.

8. Leung YY, Cheung LK. Safety of coronectomy versus excision of wisdom teeth: a randomized controlled trial. Oral Surg Oral Med Oral Pathol Oral Radiol Endod 2009;108:821—7.

9. Gleeson CF, Patel V, Kwok J, et al. Coronectomy practice. Paper 1. Technique and trouble-shooting. Br J Oral Maxillofac Surg 2012;50: 739—44.

10. Sencimen M, Ortakoglu K, Aydin C, et al. Is endodontic treatment necessary during coronectomy procedure? J Oral Maxillofac Surg 2010;68:2385—90.

11. Patel V, Gleeson CF, Kwok J, et al. Coronectomy practice. Paper 2: complications and long-term management. Br J Oral Maxillofac Surg 2013;51(4):347—52.

12. Renton T, Hankins M, Sproate C, et al. A randomized controlled clinical trial to compare the incidence of injury to the inferior alveolar nerve as a result of coronectomy and removal of mandibular third molars. Br J Oral Maxillofac Surg 2005;43: 7—12.

13. Hatano Y, Kurita K, Kuroiwa Y, et al. Clinical evaluations of coronectomy (intentional partial odontecomy) for mandibular third molars using dental computed tomography: a case-control study. J Oral Maxillofac Surg 2009;67:1806—14.

14. Leung YY, Cheung LK. Coronectomy of the lower third molar is safe within the first 3 years. J Oral Maxillofac Surg 2012;70: 1515—22.

Office Placement of Skeletal Anchorage Devices

Daniel Gill, DDS, MD [a], Stuart E. Lieblich, DMD [a,b,c],*

KEYWORDS

• Placement • Anchorage device • Skeletal • Orthodontic

KEY POINTS

• Skeletal anchorage devices enhance the versatility and expand the range of traditional orthodontic therapy.
• Rapid and reliable movement of teeth can correct some deformities that were previously only possible with invasive orthognathic surgery.
• Proper placement of devices and communication with the orthodontist are crucial to successful treatment with anchorage devices.
• Devices can be placed in the office setting in a matter of minutes without the added time, expense, and risk of treating patients in the operating room.

The placement of temporary skeletal anchorage devices is becoming increasingly common for surgeons in the office. These devices provide advantages for orthodontists and surgeons as well as patients. There are several types of skeletal anchorage device that all attempt to enhance the capabilities of traditional orthodontics.

Skeletal anchorage can provide results where traditional methods fall short. Traditional techniques involve moving a small number of teeth using a greater number of other teeth for anchorage. For difficult orthodontic movements such as distalization of molars or closure of an anterior open bite, these traditional methods provided little, if any, chance of long-term success. Other methods rely heavily on patient compliance for maintenance of elastics or headgear to provide appropriate vectors of force. Often these are unable to produce the desired movements.

Many patients and providers have opted for orthodontic camouflage of malocclusions with suboptimal results. Those who desire an optimal final result may require orthognathic surgery to correct skeletal discrepancies. However, orthognathic procedures are costly with lengthy recovery periods. They also carry considerable surgical risks of anesthesia, bleeding, nerve damage, necrosis of maxillary segments, and bad splits of the mandible. Several methods of skeletal anchorage have been developed to overcome these challenges and provide an expanded range of capabilities for the orthodontist.

Advantages of skeletal anchorage

Through the use of skeletal anchorage devices, some significant orthodontic changes can be made. Intrusion of teeth (even multiple teeth) can be accomplished quickly and easily without extruding the anchoring segment. With the intrusion of posterior teeth, the occlusal plane can be changed, leading to autorotation of the mandible, changes in lower facial height, and closure of anterior apertognathia. The procedures are simple to perform and can be done in the office with local anesthesia alone or in combination with intravenous (IV) sedation. The risks are minimal and, after a short healing time, the orthodontist can rapidly move teeth and decrease the overall orthodontic treatment time while avoiding problems with patient compliance.

Methods of skeletal anchorage

Three main devices have been used to provide anchorage. Endosseous dental implants were first used as a means of providing an immobile device for the application of force. Although dental implants can be simple to place, they are permanent and have several drawbacks compared with newer temporary devices. Dental implants are costly and require a substantial amount of bone for placement, which limits the options for appropriate placement location, and may require placement in edentulous spaces, palatal bone, or in the retromolar areas. Following placement, a delay of several weeks or months to allow for osseointegration is indicated. These drawbacks have largely been eliminated by newer temporary miniscrews and miniplates.

Placement of miniscrews

A miniscrew is a pure titanium or titanium alloy screw that is placed through mucosa directly into bone (Fig. 1) using a hand

[a] Department of Oral and Maxillofacial Surgery, University of Connecticut School of Dental Medicine, 263 Farmington Avenue, Room L-7073, Farmington, CT 06030, USA
[b] Tufts University School of Dental Medicine, One Kneeland Street, Boston, MA 02111, USA
[c] Private Practice, Avon Oral and Maxillofacial Surgery, 34 Dale Road, Suite 105, Avon, CT 06001, USA
* Corresponding author. Private Practice, Avon Oral and Maxillofacial Surgery, 34 Dale Road, Suite 105, Avon, CT 06001.
E-mail address: slieblich@avonomfs.com

Atlas Oral Maxillofacial Surg Clin N Am 21 (2013) 227-233
1061-3315/13/$ - see front matter © 2013 Elsevier Inc. All rights reserved.
http://dx.doi.org/10.1016/j.cxom.2013.05.002

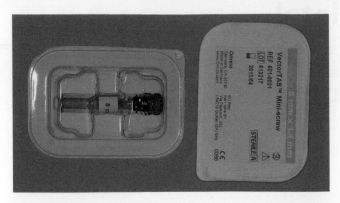

Fig. 1 Sterile packaging of 8 mm × 1.4 mm miniscrew, Ormco (Orange, CA).

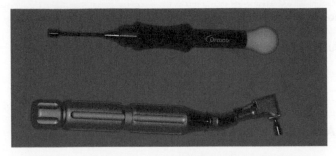

Fig. 2 Hand drivers for placement of miniscrews.

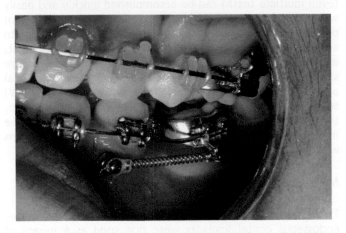

Fig. 3 Protraction of mesioangular mandibular molar using a miniscrew.

driver (Fig. 2). They are essentially a simple bone screw and can be placed in a matter of seconds by orthodontists or surgeons. Caution is needed to avoid placing screws into tooth roots, especially when placed through keratinized tissue. Placement in keratinized tissue can also limit the amount of tooth movement because of interference by the screw. This risk can be reduced by placing the miniscrews in a more apical position through nonkeratinized tissue. However, this location caries a higher risk of loosening and failure in these positions according to Cheng and colleagues.[1] Orthodontists must also use caution to avoid placing any angular moment on miniscrews to prevent turning and loosening of the screw (Fig. 3).

Placement of miniplates

Miniplates require more time and skill for placement but carry several advantages compared with miniscrews. They are often used in cases of miniscrew failure and provide a more rigid means of anchorage that can tolerate large forces. The surgeon or orthodontist can choose from a variety of designs but each plate contains a polished isthmus that extends through the mucosa to connect to the intraoral hardware. Self-drilling screws are used to secure the plate directly to bone in a variety of locations without damaging the roots of nearby teeth. The plates allow improved direct and indirect leverage and rapid movement of teeth.

Miniplate placement in the maxilla and mandible follow a few simple rules. Plates are placed apical to the tooth roots, and therefore do not interfere with tooth movement. In the maxilla, plates are placed in areas of thicker cortical bone at the buttresses of the piriform rim or zygomaticomaxillary buttress (Fig. 4). The isthmus travels through the mucosa with the attachment device positioned near or slightly apical to the dental segment and adjacent to the keratinized mucosa. The plates are malleable and easily bent to fit the bony contours.

It is not advisable to place miniplates along the anterior wall of the maxillary sinus. The bone is thin in this area and could lead to loosening of screws and loss of anchorage over time.

The mandible provides sufficient cortical bone thickness for placement of stable plates and screws in nearly any location. However, the mental nerve must be considered when planning incision design and plate placement. In the posterior regions, an incision is typically made similarly to incisions used for third molar removal or sagittal split operations for advancement or setback of the mandible. Plate placement here is far away from mandibular tooth roots and does not endanger the

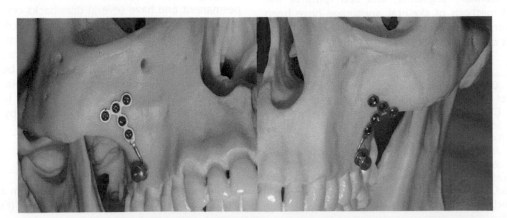

Fig. 4 (*Left*) Model showing placement of a miniplate on the zygomaticomaxillary buttress in right posterior maxilla. (*Right*) Placement in left posterior maxilla.

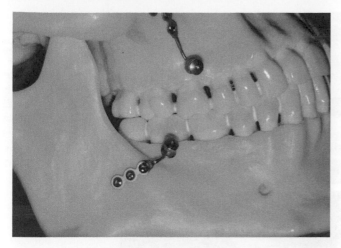

Fig. 5 Model showing option for plate placement in posterior mandible.

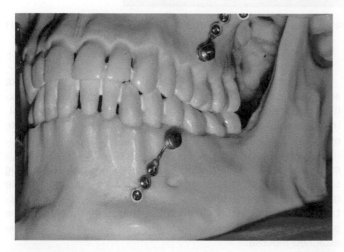

Fig. 6 Model showing plate placement in anterior mandible several millimeters anterior to the mental foramen to avoid injury to the neurovascular bundle.

inferior alveolar nerve (Fig. 5). The position allows intrusion of the posterior segment, distalization of molar teeth, and uprighting of mesioangular teeth.

Placement in the anterior mandible must avoid the mental nerve. The incision can be placed just below the mucogingival junction anterior to the premolar teeth to avoid severing the nerve within the soft tissue. Careful dissection exposes the nerve without injury for proper visualization during plate placement. Screw placement can also damage the nerve without careful consideration of anatomy of the mental nerve. Solar and colleagues[2] examined 37 preserved mandible specimens and discovered that 60% contained an anterior loop of neurovascular bundle anterior to the mental foramen. The average distance in all specimens was 1 mm with a standard deviation of 1.2 mm and a range of up to 5 mm. Other studies have confirmed the existence of an anterior loop but ranges and average distances vary. The skeletal anchorage miniplate can be placed at an angle in the anterior mandible to avoid the mental nerve and anterior loop (Fig. 6).

Clinical placement of mandibular plates

A 17-year-old boy presented with mandibular edentulous spaces caused by congenitally missing second bicuspids. The patient had previously undergone miniscrew placement for protraction of the mandibular molars. The edentulous space was unable to be closed because of premature miniscrew loosening and failure. The patient was brought in for miniplate placement under IV sedation in the office setting. A horizontal incision was made approximately 3 mm below the mucogingival junction in the area of the mandibular canine with an anterior vertical release to avoid damaging the mental nerve (Fig. 7). The incision is placed a few millimeters below the mucogingival junction to allow for ease of closure by leaving a small cuff of unattached mucosa. The plate was angled to avoid placement of screws into the anterior loop of the inferior alveolar nerve. The isthmus of the plate was bent slightly to travel transmucosally at the incision site. The plate was secured with 3 self-drilling screws and the incision closed with a few interrupted chromic sutures.

Clinical placement of maxillary plates

A 20-year-old healthy woman presents with significant anterior open bite. She was noted on examination to have contact only on her second and third molars and had notable posterior vertical maxillary excess (Fig. 8). The patient was presented

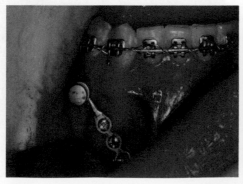
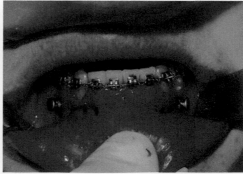

Fig. 7 (*Left*) A horizontal incision is made just below the mucogingival junction in anterior mandible with angled plate placement. (*Right*) Closure of incisions with simple chromic sutures.

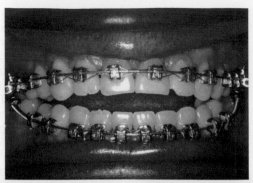

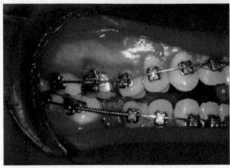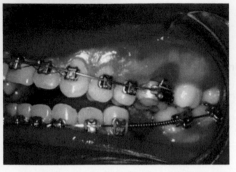

Fig. 8 (*Top*) Pretreatment view of patient with significant apertognathia. (*Lower left*) Right lateral oblique view. (*Lower right*) Left lateral oblique view.

with the option of orthognathic surgery to change the plane of occlusion and close the open bite. However, her examination also revealed a reasonable anteroposterior relationship of her maxilla and mandible along with a normal lip/tooth ratio for proper anterior maxillary esthetics. Because of these findings, we were also able to offer a reasonable alternative using maxillary miniplates. The patient was interested in a minimally invasive office-based procedure versus a conventional Le Fort I osteotomy.

In this condition, the posterior vertical excess can be reduced with intrusion of the posterior maxillary segments. This method allows autorotation of the mandible and closure of the anterior open bite. During intrusion of segments with miniplates, it is common to have buccal flaring of the involved teeth. A palatal bar should be placed to control the vector and avoid buccal flaring (Fig. 9).

The plates are placed in the posterior maxilla to take advantage of the thicker cortical bone in the zygomaticomaxillary buttress. A small horizontal incision is made a few millimeters above the mucogingival junction, again to allow ease of closure (Fig. 10).

The plates are then selected, contoured to the patient's maxillary anatomy, and secured into place with self-drilling screws (Fig. 11). Positioning is important to ensure that the isthmus travels transmucosally at the incision site in unattached mucosa, which allows the intraoral component to be positioned apical to the orthodontic wire and adjacent to the attached mucosa.

The surgical sites are irrigated with sterile saline and closed with resorbable sutures (Fig. 12). After a brief period of healing, the orthodontist can apply vertical forces to begin the intrusion process. Most patients require approximately

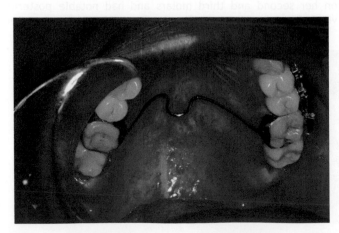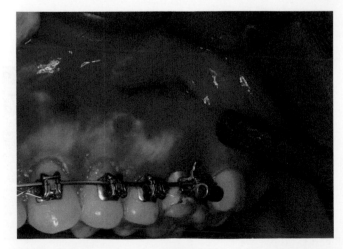

Fig. 9 Transpalatal bar to prevent buccal flaring of maxillary molar during intrusion.

Fig. 10 Incision design for plate placement in posterior maxilla just above the mucogingival junction.

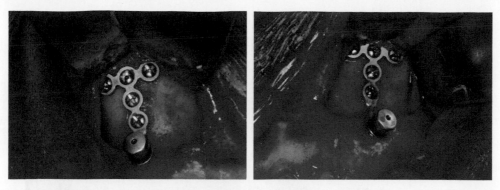

Fig. 11   Final plate placement in right posterior maxilla (*left*), and left posterior maxilla (*right*).

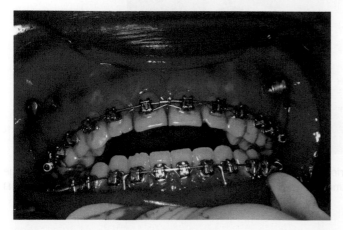

Fig. 12   Final closure of wounds with chromic gut sutures. After a short period of soft tissue healing, this patient will be ready for the application of orthodontic forces for intrusion of maxillary molars.

4 months of treatment to close an anterior open bite (Figs. 13 and 14).

Several articles have described the correction of similar open-bite deformities using mandibular miniplates to intrude lower molars, allowing for leveling the occlusal plane, auto-rotation of the mandible, and closure of anterior open bites. Intrusion of lower molars also causes buccal flaring of the intruded segment without proper orthodontic control. Flaring can be limited or eliminated by the use of a lingual bar.

Other clinical applications

Skeletal anchorage devices can be used in similar ways for the treatment of a variety of occlusal and esthetic problems. For example, miniplates can be used for the intrusion of unilateral (or bilateral) segments in preparation for prosthodontic reconstruction. With a long-standing edentulous span, the well-known phenomenon of hypereruption of the opposing

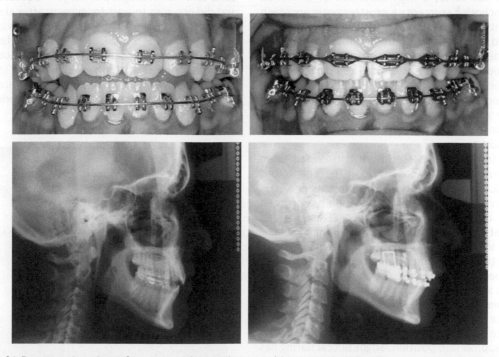

Fig. 13   (*Upper left*) Preoperative view of patient with anterior open bite treated with skeletal anchorage miniplates. (*Upper right*) Postoperative view after 4 months of treatment. (*Lower left*) Preoperative lateral cephalogram. (*Lower right*) Postoperative lateral cephalogram.

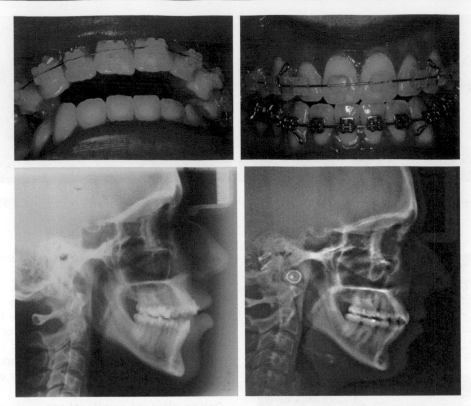

Fig. 14 (*Upper left*) Preoperative view of another patient with anterior open bite treated with skeletal anchorage miniplates to intrude upper molars. (*Upper right*) Postoperative view after 4 months of treatment. (*Lower left*) Preoperative lateral cephalogram. (*Lower right*) Postoperative lateral cephalogram.

dentition makes it difficult or impossible to place implant restorations because of lack of interocclusal space. This problem is difficult to correct by orthodontic, prosthodontic, or surgical means. Intrusion by traditional orthodontics has little chance of success but caries a high likelihood of unwanted extrusion of the anchoring segment. A prosthodontic approach requires significant reduction of tooth structure to place crowns of reduced height to level the occlusal plane. This approach also carries considerable expense for the patient and destroys natural tooth structure. A surgical approach requires an osteotomy of the segment with removal of bone, impaction of the segment, and fixation in a new position. This approach can also be costly and likely requires a general anesthetic in the operating room and a lengthy recovery period compared with skeletal anchorage.

This patient's lower right posterior dentition had been removed several years before consultation. The edentulous span was never reconstructed with dental implants or a partial denture. As a result, the opposing dentition has erupted to within a few millimeters of the lower alveolar ridge (Fig. 15). The patient now desires dental implant reconstruction of the lower posterior dentition. Using skeletal anchorage, the patient only requires orthodontic brackets on the affected segment.

A single skeletal anchorage plate is placed above the affected segment with a small horizontal incision. The plate is secured with screws and the incision is closed within minutes (Fig. 16).

After 4 months of treatment, the segment has been intruded into the appropriate position. Slight buccal flaring has occurred as a side effect of the unopposed vector of force. However, the occlusal plane has been leveled within a short time frame and without significant expense or loss of tooth

structure. The patient is now ready for implant placement and reconstruction (Fig. 17).

Another patient presents with a chief complaint of excessive gingival display (Figs. 18 and 19). This patient was not a candidate for orthognathic surgery because of his young age and did not wish to wait for surgery after skeletal maturity. An alternative, minimally invasive option was presented using miniplates. The intrusion of anterior teeth can also be accomplished with posterior maxillary plates in the zygomaticomaxillary buttress, as has been shown in several cases (as discussed earlier). With the appropriate direction of force and torque, the anterior segment can be intruded predictably.

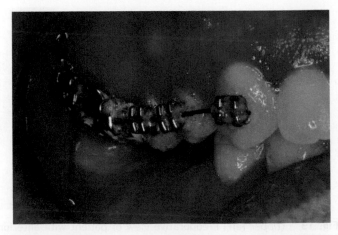

Fig. 15 Orthodontic brackets have been placed on supraerupted segment in preparation for intrusion.

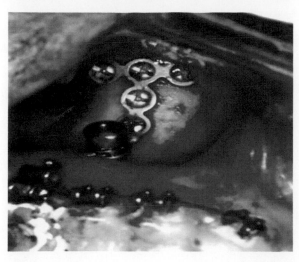

Fig. 16 A T-shaped plate has been placed in the zygomatico-maxillary buttress area and secured with 5 self-drilling screws. The oral component is positioned near the mucogingival junction.

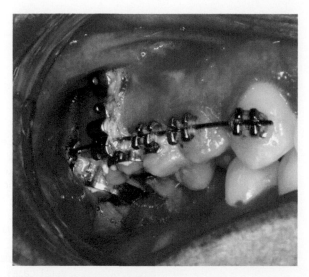

Fig. 17 Result after 4 months of intrusion forces. Slight buccal flaring of the intruded segment is noted. The mucosa is healthy and free of gingival overgrowth of the miniplate.

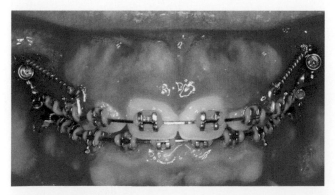

Fig. 18 Intraoral view showing skeletal anchorage plates in the posterior maxilla. After a brief period of healing, the orthodontic forces are applied.

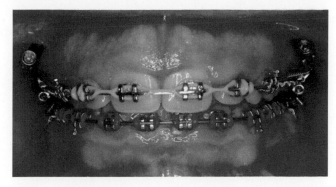

Fig. 19 Intraoral view after a few months of treatment. The patient's deep bite and gingival display have been reduced after several millimeters of intrusion of the maxillary incisors.

Summary

Temporary skeletal anchorage is a new technique that can be used to expand the office-based services provided by oral and maxillofacial surgeons. It extends the range of tooth movement for the patient and orthodontist through direct or indirect leverage. Larger forces can also be applied to the teeth to accelerate the rate of tooth movement. Temporary miniscrews can be placed in a matter of seconds with local anesthesia but must be placed with care to avoid damaging tooth roots and interfering with desired movements. Miniplates can be placed in a matter of minutes under local anesthesia with or without the use of sedation. These plates require a mucosal flap for surgical access but provide enhanced stability and can be used in cases of miniscrew failure. Both options avoid problems with unwanted anchoring tooth movements and patient compliance. They are inexpensive and do not require the period of osseointegration that is necessary after endosseous implant placement.

Over the last decade, there has been a decline in the number of orthognathic surgical procedures performed. Because of increasing health care costs and decreasing reimbursements, many patients and providers are unwilling to move forward with these lengthy and potentially risky procedures. There is a push for simpler office-based procedures that are minimally invasive and provide favorable results.

Skeletal anchorage provides versatility for the orthodontist with rapid intrusion, extrusion, protraction or retraction, correction of occlusal cants, and molar uprighting. These movements can lead to further improvements in the occlusal plane angles, position and autorotation of the mandible, closure of open bites, and reduction of excessive gingival display. Communication between the surgeon and orthodontist is crucial to the success of these procedures. They must be carefully planned and executed and require a thorough understanding of orthodontic treatment and device placement by the surgeon.

References

1. Cheng SJ, Tseng IY, Lee JJ, et al. A prospective study on the risk factors associated with failure of mini-implants used for orthodontic anchorage. Int J Oral Maxillofac Implants 2004;19:100.
2. Solar P, Ulm C, Frey G, et al. A classification of the intraosseous paths of the mental nerve. Int J Oral Maxillofac Implants 1994;9: 339—44.

Surgical Uprighting of Second Molars

Tyler Boynton, DMD [a], Stuart E. Lieblich, DMD [a,b,c],*

KEYWORDS

• Impacted teeth • Second molars • Surgical uprighting

KEY POINTS

• The second molar tooth is usually the last functional tooth to erupt and can become impacted under the distal contour of the first molar.
• Leaving the second molar in that position can damage the first molar and cause malpositioning of teeth in the opposing arch.
• Conventional orthodontic uprighting is lengthy and not always predictable, whereas surgical intervention can expedite the completion of care.

Introduction

The prevalence of impacted second molar is estimated to be approximately 3 in every 1000 patients.[1,2] They occur more frequently in the mandible than the maxilla, are usually unilateral, and are more common in females than males.[3] The primary cause can be attributed to a discrepancy in arch length. The typical pattern of resorption-apposition during mandibular development may be associated with insufficient resorption of the anterior border of the ramus. This can cause a lack of arch length causing the third molar to be situated above and behind the second molar, which prevents the natural eruption pathway of the second molar. In addition, the lack of mesial movement of the permanent first molar after exfoliation of the primary second molar can prevent eruption. A less common cause is an excess of arch length. During normal eruption, the second molar is guided into occlusion by the distal root of the first molar. When there is space between the first and second molar the second molar tends to tip mesially during eruption and the crown becomes situated beneath the height of contour of the first molar. Iatrogenic causes have also been implicated, such as bulky first molar bands (Fig. 1) and early orthodontic treatment of anterior crowding leading to insufficient space in the posterior mandible (Fig. 2).

It is essential that the treating dentist recognize and treat impacted second molar in a timely manner. Failure to do so can result in prolonged treatment times for patients undergoing orthodontic therapy and more importantly can result in loss of the first and second molar because of caries and periodontal disease. After the impacted second molar is identified, a referral should be made to a specialist who is trained in complex dentoalveolar procedures. The initial evaluation should include appropriate radiologic studies, a full medical history, a clinical examination, and a discussion with the patient and referring doctor regarding treatment options and goals.

There are many different management options that are described in the literature to treat impacted second molar. These include surgical and nonsurgical approaches. A generalization can be made that nonsurgical approaches often take longer to complete treatment; require strict patient compliance; and are technically more difficult to achieve the desired result (especially in cases of severe impactions). These techniques require that the second molar be at least partially erupted so that orthodontic appliances can be applied. To circumvent this problem, a separate surgical procedure can be performed that exposes the crown of the tooth. This not only adds another procedure, but it is difficult to keep a dry field to bond a bracket and it also causes the patient discomfort because of soft tissue overgrowth over the orthodontic appliance.

Lastly, there are several purely surgical treatment options that include the following: elective extraction of the second molar to allow eruption of the third molar; transplantation of the third molar into the second molar site; and extraction of the third molar and surgically uprighting the second molar (Fig. 3). The last of these options has been shown to be a safe and predictable procedure with excellent long-term results. The advantages of this approach are that only a single surgical procedure is necessary with a shorter overall treatment time compared with other nonsurgical options. Although there is a potential risk of root fracture and pulpal necrosis, these are exceedingly rare when the appropriate technique is used. This article describes the procedure so that the reader can achieve the same results.

Procedure

The procedure should ideally be performed when two-thirds of the second molar root is formed, which is usually between the ages of 11 and 14. If surgery is performed too soon then the tooth may be unstable and may shift in position. If performed too late then there is risk of root fracture and possible disruption of blood supply leading to pulpal necrosis.[4]

[a] Department of Oral and Maxillofacial Surgery, University of Connecticut School of Dental Medicine, 263 Farmington Avenue, Farmington, CT 06030, USA
[b] Tufts University School of Dental Medicine, One Kneeland Street, Boston, MA 02111, USA
[c] Private Practice, Avon Oral and Maxillofacial Surgery, 34 Dale Road, Suite 105, Avon, CT 06001, USA
* Corresponding author. Avon Oral and Maxillofacial Surgery, Private Practice, 34 Dale Road, Suite 105, Avon, CT 06001.
E-mail address: slieblich@avonomfs.com

Atlas Oral Maxillofacial Surg Clin N Am 21 (2013) 235-237
1061-3315/13/$ - see front matter © 2013 Elsevier Inc. All rights reserved.
http://dx.doi.org/10.1016/j.cxom.2013.05.001

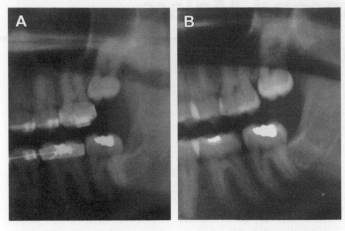

Fig. 1 (*A*) Impacted maxillary second molar caused by over-contoured molar band. (*B*) Maxillary second molar eruption after removal of molar band.

In the authors' experience, a higher rate of postoperative infection has been noted anecdotally and therefore a single preoperative dose of oral or intravenous antibiotics is recommended. The armamentarium is essentially the same for surgical exposure and extraction of third molars. An intrasulcular incision should be made from the distobuccal line angle of the first molar and extended posteriorly toward the external oblique ridge (Fig. 4). A full-thickness mucoperiosteal flap is then raised to expose the second and third molar (if present).

A surgical handpiece with a round or fissure bur is used to expose the third molar, which can then be sectioned and extracted. The handpiece is then used to remove bone distal to the second molar and a buccal trough is made so that the

cementoenamel junction is exposed. Great care must be taken during this step to avoid contact with the cementum and periodontal ligament fibers because this may cause external root resorption.

A straight elevator is then inserted on the mesial of the second molar and the handle is then turned toward the tooth so that the upper edge of the blade is just inferior to the height of contour. A steady downward force is then applied along the handle at the same time, which elevates the tooth distally. It is important that the surgeon use steady and gentle force to prevent root fracture. If the surgeon encounters difficulty uprighting the second molar then additional distal bone may be removed with a handpiece. Once the crown of the second molar clears the height of contour of the first molar, the patient is instructed to bite down gently to ensure that the molar is just below the occlusal plane to prevent occlusal trauma. In most cases, the second molar is stable because it is wedged between distal bone and the crown of the first molar. An intact lingual and buccal plate prevents the tooth from migrating bucally or lingually. No additional autogenous bone or bone substitutes are needed to stabilize the tooth and it is rare that additional methods are needed to stabilize the tooth. The site should be irrigated with copious amounts of normal saline and then closed with sutures. The attached gingiva should be kept intact and positioned appropriately to ensure a healthy periodontal environment for the newly positioned second molar. An immediate postoperative Panorex is recommended for baseline documentation. The patient is instructed to follow the standard postoperative instructions for third molar removal and is also given an irrigating syringe to remove food debris that becomes trapped between the first and second molar. Follow-up includes a 1-week postoperative appointment and then another appointment in 6 months for a repeat Panorex.

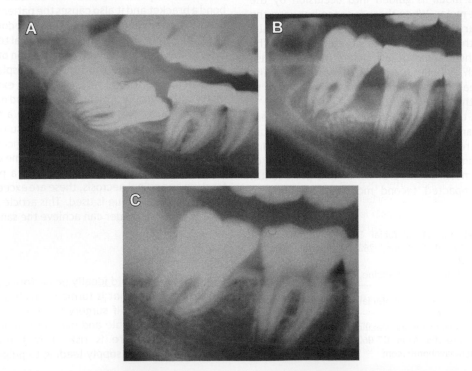

Fig. 2 (*A*) Impacted mandibular second molar. (*B*) Immediate postoperative view of mandibular second molar surgical uprighting. (*C*) Fourteen months postoperative view of uprighted second molar with adequate vertical bone fill between the first and second molar.

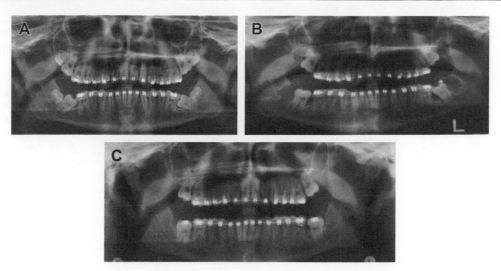

Fig. 3 (*A*) Preoperative Panorex of bilateral impacted mandibular second molar. (*B*) Immediate postoperative Panorex after extraction of third molars and surgical uprighting of mandibular second molar. (*C*) One-year postoperative Panorex demonstrating adequate bone fill and no periapical pathology.

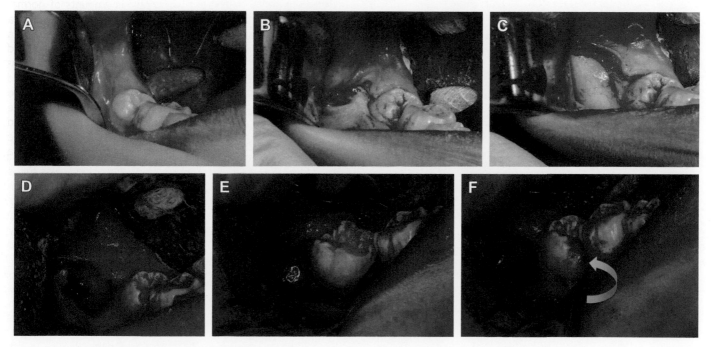

Fig. 4 (*A*) Preoperative photograph showing impacted second molar. (*B*) Intrasulcular incision with distal-oblique release. (*C*) Surgical exposure of anterior border of ramus. (*D*) Extraction of third molar. (*E*) Uprighting of second molar using a straight elevator. (*F*) Rotation of straight elevator toward tooth with downward motion of the handle.

Summary

The surgical uprighting of second molar is a fast, reliable, and predictable method of correcting second molar impactions. Long-term follow-up shows that there is a low rate of peri-apical pathology, root fracture, pulpal necrosis, and peri-odontal bone defects. By following these simple techniques, the surgeon is able to effectively treat second molar impactions with a low complication rate.

References

1. Grover PS, Norton L. The incidence of unerupted permanent teeth and related clinical cases. Oral Surg Oral Med Oral Pathol 1985;59:420—59.
2. Yehoshua S, Borell G, Nahlieli O, et al. Second molar impactions. Angle Orthod 1999;68:173—8.
3. Frank C. Treatment options for impacted teeth. J Am Dent Assoc 2000;131:623—32.
4. Dessner S. Surgical uprighting of second molars: rationale and technique. Oral Maxillofac Surg Clin North Am 2002;14:201—12.

Moving?

Make sure your subscription moves with you!

To notify us of your new address, find your **Clinics Account Number** (located on your mailing label above your name), and contact customer service at:

Email: journalscustomerservice-usa@elsevier.com

800-654-2452 (subscribers in the U.S. & Canada)
314-447-8871 (subscribers outside of the U.S. & Canada)

Fax number: 314-447-8029

Elsevier Health Sciences Division
Subscription Customer Service
3251 Riverport Lane
Maryland Heights, MO 63043

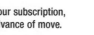

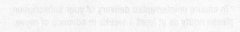

Printed and bound by CPI Group (UK) Ltd, Croydon, CR0 4YY

03/10/2024

01040378-0019